Rainbow

OF HOPE

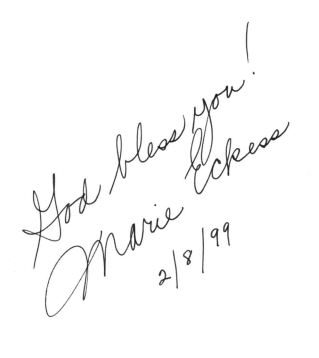

God bless you!

Marie Eckess

2/8/99

Rainbow
OF HOPE

Marie Eckess, Ph.D.

WINEPRESS 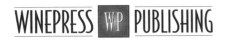 PUBLISHING

Scripture quotations are from the New King James version of the Holy Bible by Thomas Nelson, Inc. Copyright 1985

Non-scriptural quotations are from the International Dictionary of Thoughts, J.G. Ferguson Publishing Co. Copyright 1969

ISBN 1-57921-157-7
Library of Congress Catalog Card Number: 98-88569

DEDICATION

To Mother and Aunt Marie

Devoted sisters, whose faith in God was the bedrock of their strong characters. Their lives reflected perseverance, honesty, compassion, generosity, forgiveness, and hope. Our families were encircled by the love of these courageous women.

To my husband, Bill

Whose abiding faith, devotion, support, and encouragement continues to provide a calm in the midst of life's storms. Bill is my best friend, the love of my life.

ACKNOWLEDGMENTS

I HONOR MY WOMEN FRIENDS—all wives and mothers—whose diligence, truth, and prayerful generosity guided me as they reviewed the rough drafts that gave birth to *Rainbow of Hope*. Their patient commitment to our mutual goal of providing this book of hope, awareness, and faith, speaks volumes of their character. These women are encouragers. These are women I love and admire:

- Eileen Daniels: A born caregiver, my kindred-spirit, beloved cousin

- Gloria Fahey: Nurturing neighbor and community activist

- Michelle Garber: Registered nurse

- Lyn Hagopian: Marriage and Family Therapist

- Marilyn Tift: Small business owner

I honor Stella A. Chavos, Certified Pedorthist, owner of Newport Center Orthopedic, Inc., who shows sensitivity and compassion in meeting a woman's need for a prosthesis after the mastectomy. Stella understands pain and loss because she has osteoporosis, but her smile is the first thing I always see, reflecting her positive attitude.

I honor the 100 interviewees who shared their intimate details of coping with breast cancer. They are the very essence of this book.

I honor the staff and associates of WinePress Publishing for their creative dedication to making *Rainbow of Hope* a reality in print.

CONTENTS

PREFACE

TWENTY-FIVE YEARS AGO, I made a promise to share the courageous stories of seventy women and our journey with breast cancer. Today, I am prepared to keep my promise to relive and relate those shared moments of individual experiences that represent our trials of endurance and our victory.

Our story begins with a question we struggled to answer—the same question I see women struggling with today. Why do some women accept the pressure of believing that breasts or breast size defines who they are? Our culture attempts to define us through breast norms and standards. These dictated measurements may vary over time but have exerted painful influence upon a woman's identity.

The response has been to push up, push out, rouge, oil, and/or expose what we have for approval. Small-breasted women find they do not have as much to push, pull, or tug; medium-breasted women may also be dissatisfied. Both often seek cosmetic breast enlargement. Large-breasted women, happy with their size, either revel in exposing their breasts or are too shy to follow the fashion of the day and, if unhappy, seek surgical breast reduction.

Our society continues to decree whether breasts are suitably voluptuous, too small, or too large, while the advertising world offers padding, ointment, and Wonder Bras. Cosmetic research offers silicone injection as the ultimate solution for beauty.

Confused women walk our land, either satisfied or agonized in the belief that their breast measurement is the true reflection of their stature as worthy individuals.

In shadows, threatening male desire and female vanity, lurks this fallacy's greatest rival: breast cancer, two words that forever change a woman. Is it any wonder that so many women are devastated when they lose one or both breasts to cancer?

We absorb this misconception in our childhood. Children long to grow up and emulate their parents. Breasts are related to sex, and boys and girls observe that adult women have larger breasts. Many of us can remember the excitement of getting that first bra—in the past, a hand-me-down from an older sister or cousin and considered a precious gift—a sign of becoming a woman. Today, preteens prize training-bras for the same reason.

Back in the thirties, little girls danced in the rain with brothers and cousins, wearing only panty underwear. Mom rushed out and told them to come in and put on a top because they were too old to play in front of boys without one. Growing up begins to cause inner conflict because of losing a precious freedom, the freedom of innocence. Breasts begin to take on an importance that torments, because the commotion over a bare chest is not understood.

Every girl wants to belong, to be a part of the group. Youngsters look around and see girlfriends with growing breasts and accept this. One day, however, some girls grow larger breasts and suffer teasing because of their "problem." Little boys giggle as they make fun of "large boobs" and accuse little girls of being sexually loose, because everyone knows that large breasts accompany promiscuity. Boys also taunt flat-chested girls who have only "fried eggs."

Parents tell children to stand up straight in order to have good posture, but many young girls slump over in shame because of their "large boobs" or "fried eggs." Who needs that? Girls with medium-sized breasts seem to have the best posture around.

Thus, the existence of breasts and the size of our breasts begins to define who we are and what makes us sexy and desirable.

We seventy women who share our experiences with you, have had similar identity struggles and have been caught in the same snare of dictated norms and standards. However, for us there has been one major difference: we have had to redefine ourselves after developing breast cancer—not an easy task when faced with the continued onslaught of social norms, advertising, male reactions, and our own struggles with self-esteem.

If it is true that our breasts play such a large part in defining us and our significance, then as victims of breast cancer, who we are remains in some operating room. But some of us reject this notion, knowing that we are much more than our breasts. We are dedicated to living every day as an affirmation of our capacity for a positive, contributing life, because inwardly we are whole.

Newport Beach, California   Marie Eckess, Ph.D.
September, 1998

INTRODUCTION

I RECALL AWAKENING IN THE HOSPITAL recovery room on September 24, 1974—five days before my forty-third birthday. My first remembrance was of a nurse dressed in green, bending over my bed and asking, "Why aren't you crying? Don't you know what they have done to you?" I thought, *What a fearsome thing for her to say.* I had adjusted to the knowledge that I might awaken without a breast, but her face and voice reflected personal horror.

As I lay in the hospital bed for seven days, that nurse's comment continued to haunt me. Why was she so terrified? I had accepted my loss better than she, and I felt saddened at her having burdened me with her fear. I had enough of my own personal health concerns to overcome. After previous non-cancerous surgeries, I had awakened to the sweet, loving voices of family members and friends, but this time felt cheated by the intrusion of a stranger's voice so filled with her expectations of my loss.

In the days and months that followed my hospitalization, the fear of cancer reflected in the faces and voices of loved ones. They expressed sincere concern, but their fear seemed to all but paralyze some, as though extending their hands while standing remotely at a distance in order to prevent cancer from happening to them.

I found comfort in prayer and in the promise of the Twenty-third Psalm—"The Lord is my shepherd . . ."—and promised myself three things. First, I would not allow myself to diminish because of the loss of a breast. Second, I would not consider my body ugly, only changed. Third, I would verbally and prayerfully fight this disease, seeking and sharing knowledge of cancer with the intent of comforting, encouraging, and informing other women who might also be victims of this silent attacker.

Refusal to listen, learn, and take necessary action against cancer constitutes crimes of silence and apathy. Despite extensive research over forty years, we still know little about cancer as individuals and as a society. The very mention of the word numbs the mind. Why do people fear cancer even more than a heart attack? I have concluded that the answer lies in the fact that the subject of cancer has been a secretive topic in the past, just as in former times, the retarded child was locked away in the closet and never discussed. Although public awareness of the struggle of the retarded child today has improved, few people acknowledge the struggle of cancer, let alone discuss it. Silence will not cure. Silence is no longer acceptable.

The loss of a breast in our youth-oriented culture is particularly daunting. It is not in vogue to be old, wrinkled, or fat, let alone maimed. The prevailing mentality is that we must stay young at all costs, even into our eighties. This search for youth denies the pleasure of each decade of life. We cease to look for the beauty within each stage, and instead become frustrated, angered, and dissatisfied with our looks and ourselves in general.

We imprison ourselves by these attitudes and fears. This shell, our body, will deteriorate, as does every part of nature in its own time. By refusing to accept this truth, we deny the fact that death is a natural process. Are we allowing fear to eat away at our intellect, our spirits, and our courage?

Method of Research

With the encouragement of a writer-friend in 1974, a staff member of the *Daily Pilot* newspaper was contacted and wrote a feature article about my intended book related to mastectomy. We put out a request for volunteers who'd had such breast cancer surgery to participate by agreeing to personal interviews.

The Journal and the *Huntington Beach Independent* newspapers also published articles. The Orange County Division of the American Cancer Society assisted me by receiving phone messages and written correspondence from women willing to participate.

Seventy women volunteered, ages twenty-seven to seventy-nine. All known forms of mastectomy surgery had been performed, from within six weeks to twenty-two years prior to interviewing. The majority had lost one breast; nine had lost both. Participants included married, divorced, single, and widowed women from many walks of life, including an artist-sculptor, college students, business executives, entrepreneurs, a professional cook, teachers, nurses, homemakers, saleswomen, waitresses, secretaries, typists, an insurance underwriter, school administrators, clerks, socialites, and a laundry worker. In several instances, husbands and adult children shared their thoughts as well.

Although the volunteers resided in Orange County, California, several had their surgery prior to moving to the state. In the book, as promised, I use no real names. Also, ages of the women are noted as in the following example: (27/27). The first number is the age at the time of surgery; the second number is the age at time of interview. One volunteer, Amy (57/59), a cerebral palsy victim confined to a wheelchair since childhood, could communicate with me only through her typewriter and caregiver.

Within six weeks of my surgery, I began taping interviews, either at my home or at theirs. Some women chose telephone interviews, feeling too ill to leave their homes. Beth (40/51), who died before our interview, had told her husband of her desire to participate, so he volunteered to speak on her behalf. In addition to these seventy women with mastectomies, another thirty women and men approached me, wanting to share their experiences with breast cancer that had struck their families or friends, and I took written notes. Selected detailed interviews are quoted throughout this book, as they best reflect and articulate the thoughts of all one hundred participants.

Fifty-three women participated in taped interviews and answered questions regarding the following:

1. Family history of cancer
2. How cancer was discovered
3. Reaction upon discovery
4. Type of physician contacted
5. Mammography used
6. Time lapse from discovery to biopsy
7. Family reactions
8. Personal knowledge of cancer prior to mastectomy
9. How doctor described mastectomy and alternatives
10. Radiation/chemotherapy discussion prior to surgery
11. How surgeon was chosen
12. Extent of surgery and self-understanding of surgery
13. Possession of pathology report
14. Any therapy during hospital stay
15. Reaction of hospital staff
16. Remembrance of hospital stay (visitors, physical, psychological)
17. Adjustment at home (self, family, friends)
18. Ability to use arms
19. Adjustments upon returning to work
20. Reaction to seeing incision (self, husband, family)
21. Entire process of choosing and purchasing prosthesis/implants
22. All aspects of treatment after mastectomy
23. Follow-up examinations
24. What helped the most to accept/adjust to cancer and mastectomy
25. Any suggestions to women needing breast cancer treatment
26. Reaction to literature and media on breast cancer
27. Any suggestions to husbands, physicians, nurses, etc.
28. Any unanswered questions.

The content of this book does not pretend to answer all questions. I encourage women to raise their own questions and take responsibility for their own bodies and lives. Our main goal focuses on reaching out a hand of encouragement to those of you who may personally have breast cancer, or who have a loved one with this disease. There is hope!

Knowledge and faith turn into fighting tools. Not only do we owe it to ourselves to become better informed, but we also owe it to every living person and their unborn children. Women with breast cancer—living and dead—have contributed positively to the knowledge and faith needed in our defense against cancer.

I promised seventy women in 1974–1975 that I would write this book as a source of hope and encouragement to other women, their families, children, and caregivers. You may justifiably ask why it took me so long to keep my promise. The death of women shortly before and after their interviews had an extremely painful effect on me. Each time I began to write, I would dissolve into tears. Hearing their voices and laughter on the tapes further wounded my heart. Over the years, I have prayed they will understand and forgive my delay.

We must always learn to trust in God's perfect timing. In November 1995, I miraculously survived a double brain aneurysm unrelated to cancer. I began rereading my Bible, which firmly reminded me that God says we are to keep our word when once we've given it. I cannot respect myself if I do not do so. With the continued help of God, and out of gratitude and love for Him and these seventy women, this book will be a testimony that my word is my bond.

We lovingly offer you this gift of our knowledge, with the prayer that you will benefit from what we have experienced. May this book honor all who, for the purpose of helping others, shared and entrusted me with their innermost feelings. God bless each of them, their families, and you.

My heart leaps up when I behold
A rainbow in the sky:
So was it when my life began;
So is it now I am a man;
So be it when I shall grow old,
Or let me die.
The child is father of the man;
And I could wish my days to be
Bound each to each by natural piety.

—WILLIAM WORDSWORTH
English poet (1770–1850)

1

LOOK FOR THE RAINBOWS

"Be thou the rainbow to the storms of life,
the evening beam that smiles the clouds away,
and tints tomorrow with prophetic ray!"
—Lord Byron
English poet (1788–1824)

A RAINBOW MEANS DIFFERENT THINGS to different people. "The gracious thing, made of tears and light," wrote English poet Samuel Taylor Coleridge (1771–1834). English Anglican clergyman Charles Caleb Colton (1780?–1832) called it "that smiling daughter of the storm." To me, the rainbow is a promise of God's eternal love, reminding me that I was not alone nor forgotten in my struggle against breast cancer.

Thus, I view the rainbow as a perfect analogy to tell you of my well-remembered impressions of seventy women with mastectomies, and to offer you my personal thoughts about my journey and survival these past twenty-five years.

As we emerged from our cancer storms, some women were emotionally and psychologically unable to see a promising future without their breasts. A few spoke of wanting to die or commit suicide. Cancer had attacked us as individuals, and as individuals we had to choose our response.

Faith through prayer helped me and others to find God's rainbow of hope, and each woman viewed it from her own mastectomy experience. However, not all the women looked for the rainbow.

I have always eagerly searched the horizon after a rainstorm or shower, hoping to find a magical rainbow with all of its beautiful spectrum of colors. Sometimes a double rainbow appears, and I am captivated and absorbed by the beauty of these moments. When a rainbow pattern of light reveals itself to me, a sense of joy and wonder and renewal overtakes me as I see this splendid partnership between rain and sun and God. My experience with and survival of breast cancer can be compared to the storms and sunlight that produce magnificent rainbows.

As a child, I often wondered if the rainbow observed us as well, and considered what a raindrop would say if it could speak. Isn't it wonderful that no matter how old we become, or what tragedy befalls us, we can still nurture that imaginative child that lives within us! A mastectomy is such a tragedy, but our attitude can help us rise above it.

As a brief illustration, I present a trusting, imaginative raindrop with a very positive self-image in order to tell you why I do not relate to women who define themselves by their breasts to such a degree that they see future life as hopeless and futile without them; nor do I relate to the few who live with the thoughts of suicide and wanting to die. I have always known that I am more than my breasts.

I Am a Trusting Raindrop

I love being a member of a family of raindrops. God considers each of us important and sends us to help replenish and serve all living things when we descend to earth.

My raindrop family takes pleasure in observing the benefits our hard work produces: the laughter of children as they play in our water puddles; the sweet fragrance from grass and flowers we nourish; the sparking, clean streets we carefully wash; the singing of birds as they bathe in our pools; the contentment of animals as they drink at our water's edge; and the prayers of human beings thanking God for our gift of life. We raindrops are grateful for our place in God's universe.

But we are sad when too many of us fall to earth at the same time with storms that cause floods and destruction. No raindrop I know ever volunteers to be destructive. We don't want to cause anyone to cry or to see anyone harmed.

My rainbow family often discusses our sorrow, and most of us accept the reality that there are situations beyond our control and which we simply do not understand. Nevertheless, we know our duty is to become the best raindrops possible, trusting God for the result He desires.

Our schools teach us that a typical raindrop is spherical. Those of us who are large will help the sun produce bright rainbows, and if we are small, our rainbows will have overlapping colors that appear almost white.

We raindrops work very hard with the sun to make a variety of bows for you humans to enjoy: primary, secondary, and tertiary rainbows; fogbows; and colored arcs that are formed in sea spray or in the spray of waterfalls, garden hoses, or lawn sprinklers. Your joy in finding us is our reward!

It is not easy for us to come to earth and make a rainbow. Sometimes our spherical shapes are shattered because of collision with other raindrops, or flattened by the natural drop as we fall in the air. Our changed shapes will limit our ability to help the sun reflect brightly colored rainbows, but our teachers tell us that no matter the shape of our droplets, we are all of value and can do our part for God. But some raindrops can't or won't accept this truth.

For example, my sister raindrop has always planned and longed to become part of a primary rainbow—the kind appearing after a heavy rainfall and creating a brilliant bow that spans the entire horizon. Human folklore tells of a pot of gold waiting to be claimed where the ends of this rainbow seem to touch the earth. My sister raindrop insists upon being in the red arc at the top, because it has a longer wavelength than violet, which appears at the bottom. She needs to be seen.

My sister raindrop has never wanted to hear about the joys of being a part of God's other endeavors. Now that her shape has been changed because of a collision with another raindrop, she becomes angry when anyone tries to bring up the subject of positive alternatives. One of the first things we learn in our schools is that, in order to make a rainbow, we must accept the sun's rays into our shapes, and then we must work hard to bend and reflect the colors that make a rainbow.

However, my sister raindrop refuses to bend, even when it is in her own best interest to do so. In this, she reminds me of many humans I have observed who never seem to be satisfied with who they are or what they have in life. When tragedy comes, they see only negatives, because they will not bend toward new possibilities. Do they not realize that their negative reflections cannot bring beauty into the lives of others?

As a trusting raindrop, I know that if my shape becomes shattered or flattened as I fall to earth, God will still love and use me in ways that are pleasing to Him. Therein lies my joy and gratitude.

I pray that God allows me to become a part of any rainbow of His choosing. No two rainbows are alike, and as with humans, we raindrops are a mixture of many sizes and shapes. No matter what my shape is like, I want the privilege of helping people find joy in their lives.

After a shower or storm, please look for me on the horizon, as one day I may well be in a rainbow, looking and smiling back at you, reminding you that God's unconditional love is eternal!

"A smile is a whisper of a laugh."
—Anonymous

"Trust in God does not supersede the employment of prudent means on our part. To expect God's protection while we do nothing is not to honor but to tempt providence."

—PASQUIER QUESNEL
French Theologian (1634–1719)

2

EARLY DETECTION
SAVES LIVES

"Choose life, that both thou and thy seed may live."
—*Deuteronomy 30:19*

WE WOMEN WHO SHARE OUR STORIES and journeys in this book are no different than you in our feelings and emotions upon hearing the words *breast cancer.* Our experiences confirm the attitudes of denial, fear, and procrastination. These same attitudes continue today and keep many women from learning more about how to protect themselves from breast cancer. The encouraging and hopeful reality is that breast cancer has a very high cure rate if caught in its beginning stages.

What Is Breast Cancer?

"Cancer is classified by the part of the body in which it develops, by its appearance under the microscope, and the results of laboratory tests. Since cancer is not a single disease, each type of cancer behaves differently, and it also responds differently to various types of treatment. This makes it very important to treat each cancer and each cancer patient individually."[1]

Normal cells divide and grow in an organized manner, but cancer cells expand out of control. This attack on normal tissue can grow and spread, and if not controlled, death occurs. Most types of cancer cells create a mass called a "malignant tumor." Metastasis occurs if cells break away from the original tumor and are spread by the lymph system or the bloodstream to other parts of the body, where the cancer begins anew.

Many breast tumors such as fibroadenomas or papillomas are not cancerous. These benign tumors usually are contained in one area (in situ), are limited in growth, and are not considered life threatening.

Early detection is vital. If we take responsibility for our own bodies and lives by learning all we can about breast cancer and early detection methods, we can be among those who survive.

Three-Step Early Detection Program

Early detection of any abnormality in the breast provides us with the opportunity to seek immediate medical help. The practice of breast self-examination (BSE) allows us to stay in tune with our body by checking monthly for any changes that might develop. Regularly scheduled clinical breast examinations also add to our chances for early detection and survival.

The American Cancer Society has developed a three-step early detection program:

- Breast self-exam: Every woman aged twenty or older, every month.
- Clinical breast exam: Ages twenty to thirty-nine, every three years; after age forty, every year.
- Mammography: All women aged forty and older.[2]

The Monthly Practice of Breast Self-Examination (BSE)

The American Cancer Society guidelines advise that the best time to do BSE is about a week after your menstrual period or on a select day that's easy to remember. Follow the three-step process outlined below:

1. Lie down with your right shoulder on a pillow or folded towel, and put your right hand behind your head. With

the fingers of your left hand flat, press down on your right breast using a circular motion. Feel for any lumps or thickenings. Do the same on your left side. Also, squeeze each nipple and the area around the nipples gently checking for any clear or bloody discharge.

2. Examine your breasts in front of a mirror, first standing and then with your hands in the air, followed by your hands pressing down on your hips. Look for changes in size or shape, dimpling or puckering, or unusual changes in the appearance or position of the nipple.

3. You may also want to perform BSE in the shower, where fingers glide easily over wet, soapy skin. Keep your fingers flat and move your hand over your right breast while holding your right arm in the air. Then do the same on the left side. Contact your physician immediately if you find any abnormality.[3]

Our Breast Self-Examination Experiences in 1974–1975

The majority of the women interviewed either haphazardly examined their breasts, or not at all. Some lumps were found accidentally by the woman, by her husband, or as in one case, by a fiancé. Most lumps, however, were discovered by doctors during clinical examinations.

Kitty (29/31) never practiced breast self-examination, even though her maternal grandmother died of breast cancer, and her mother experienced the loss of both breasts within a five-year interval. "It was always in the back of my mind that I would get cancer, but not at the age of twenty-nine. I didn't examine myself, because I didn't expect to get it so young. I think that if I had reached thirty-four or forty, I would have started to examine myself on a regular basis. My mother and grandmother got it for the first time when they were in their fifties." Kitty had a radical mastectomy at the age of twenty-nine and died at the age of thirty-one, shortly after our interview, leaving two young daughters ages three and nine.

The husband of Opal (34/56) found the lump accidentally as they sat on their couch. "I thought it wouldn't happen to me. That is something I just didn't anticipate. I simply refused to entertain the idea." Opal had a radical mastectomy at the age of thirty-four and survived to tell of her experience twenty-two years later.

The fiancé of Tressa (33/33) insisted that the lump he discovered be examined immediately by a doctor. "I joked about it and told him my breasts are lumpy because they are large and have a lot of tissue. I preferred to think there was nothing." At the age of thirty-three, Tressa had a double radical mastectomy in 1975 and happily married her loving fiancé that year.

Becky (51/51) practiced breast self-examination. "I was pretty confident. I am a nurse by profession and have been teaching breast self-examination for eight years with the American Cancer Society. I would only have myself to blame, because I know how to examine my breasts monthly and am extremely familiar with the 'geography' of my breasts. I would come out of this with my life, and that is all I really cared about."

Our Clinical Examination Experiences

We told our doctors of concern about breast distortions, such as a pucker, dimple, or swelling; black-and-blue skin discoloration; nipples that burned, were inverted, or secreted a nonclear discharge; or pain or tingling sensation when cysts changed and enlarged. Some of us had fibrocystic breast disease, also called chronic cystic mastitis, which is the most common nonmalignant breast disorder in women. Sixty-one women had single mastectomies, and nine had double mastectomies.

Based upon our experiences, I question the wisdom of limiting women ages twenty to thirty-nine to a clinical exam only once every three years. Ten of the seventy women in 1974–1975 were in this age group. Their ages were twenty-seven, twenty-nine, thirty-two, thirty-three, thirty-four, thirty-eight, and thirty-nine (four women). Often it was the physicians who found lumps by clinical breast examinations. Double mastectomies were performed on Tressa (33/33) and Kitty (29/31) who died at the age of thirty-one.

We encourage this age group to have clinical breast exams every year, not every three years. Shame on our society if we don't extend this encouragement and provide insurance coverage. If our government can find funds to pay for birth control in foreign countries, funds surely can be found to spare the lives of young American women from cancer.

Kitty (29/31) would agree if she were alive to speak for herself. After all, she left two daughters who today are twenty-seven and thirty-three.

Statistics and Risk Factors for Breast Cancer

Presently, we do not know what causes cancer, and there is no known way to prevent breast cancer. Extensive research continues internationally.

Statistical Factors

The American Cancer Society estimates that "in 1998, there will [have been] some 178,700 women diagnosed as having invasive breast cancer in the United States, of whom about 43,900 deaths will occur. Breast cancer is the leading cause of death among women aged forty to fifty-five. Women aged twenty to twenty-nine account for only 0.3 percent of diagnosed breast cancers. About 77 percent of women with breast cancer are over the age of fifty. White women (113.1 per 100,000) are slightly more likely to develop breast cancer than African-American women (101.0 per 100,000). Under the age of forty-five, African-American women (31.2 per 100,000) are more likely to develop breast cancer and more likely to die of breast cancer, compared to white women (26.00 per 100,000)."[4]

The University Health Quarterly of New Jersey suggests, "Each day this year alone, 500 women are presented with the diagnosis. That's one new case about every three minutes."[5]

Risk Factors

The University Health Quarterly of New Jersey also describes age, family history, and reproductive history as the three dominant risk factors associated with breast cancer.[6]

1. **Age.** The odds go up as you grow older. For example, only 1 out of 500 women in their thirties will have breast cancer. By the time they are forty-five to fifty, the incidence goes up to 1 out of 50. And for women in their eighties, breast cancer will strike 1 out of 9.

Our age risk factor. Statistically, our age risk factor represents a significant comparison to current research provided. Out of 95 percent of the women interviewed who disclosed their ages, 74 percent were in the forty-and-above range. Twenty-one percent had mastectomies between the ages of twenty-seven and thirty-nine. Two had double mastectomies—one at age twenty-seven and the other at age thirty-three.

Thirty-six percent had mastectomies in our forties, including myself. Three had double mastectomies, one losing her breasts six years apart, at ages forty-one and forty-seven. Thirty-eight percent of us had mastectomies between the ages of fifty-one and seventy-eight. Three of these women had double mastectomies, with one losing her breasts two years apart, at ages forty-nine and fifty-one. (Five percent of the women did not disclose their ages.)

2. **Family history.** This predisposing factor is most significant if your mother was diagnosed before menopause or if both your mother and sister had breast cancer. A family history of breast cancer is the strongest known risk factor, yet it's missing from up to 80 percent of diagnosed cancers.

Our family history risk factor. Just twenty-one women in our group had a family history of cancer. Of those, only Esther (44/57) had a mother and sister with breast cancer. Since cancer has a long history of silence, Ethel (41/47) wasn't sure who may have had cancer in her family. "They just didn't talk about those kinds of things."

Known family females with a form of cancer were grand-mothers, mothers, aunts, great-aunts, and sisters. Of these, some had died from cancer of the lungs, uterus, thyroid, brain, rectum, and breast. Several had survived breast cancer. Known family males with a form of cancer included a son, fathers, grandfathers, uncles, and brothers. Of these, death had occurred from cancer of the lungs, prostate, liver, kidneys, throat, colon, stomach, lymph glands, leukemia, and rectum.

Bertha (64/64) had the most cancer in her family history. Her mother died of lymph cancer, her father of throat cancer, her maternal aunt of breast and uterus cancer, and her maternal uncle from prostate cancer. Jan (32/32) had a fraternal aunt who'd had breast cancer but who had lived into her eighties. Of the nine women with double mastectomies, five had no family history of cancer. The sister of Beatrice (54/55) had died of breast cancer, and lung cancer had taken her father. Agnes (48/58) reported liver and rectum cancer on both sides of her family. The mother of Olivia (45/54) had cancer of the cervix in 1954 and was still living twenty years later. The mother of Daisy (59/62) had died of thyroid cancer, and her father had died of colon cancer. Kitty (29/31) had a family history of both grandmothers dying of cancer and her mother surviving a double mastectomy, with surgeries performed five years apart.

3. **Reproductive history.** Early menstruation, late menopause, and delayed or no child-bearing carry slightly increased risks.

Our reproductive history risk factor. The mothers of our group had a combined total of 120 children, ranging from one to seven children per family. Eight women had borne three children; seven, four children; one, five children; three, six children; and one, seven children. There were sixty-one sons and fifty-nine daughters. Eight of us had borne no children. All of us had mastectomies.

The complexity of cancer and statistics is evident in that although my experience most closely parallels the reproductive history risk factor of being childless, I have survived these past twenty-five years. Kitty (29/31), who bore two children, died at the age of thirty-one.

Additional Risk-Factor Findings

The American Cancer Society designates fourteen additional risk factors associated with breast cancer, which include: (1) a personal history of breast cancer; (2) previous breast biopsy; (3) estrogen replacement therapy; (4) higher education or socioeconomic level; (5) lifestyle choices; (6) alcohol; (7) smoking; (8) high-fat diets and being overweight; (9) exercise; (10) oral contraceptives; (11) environmental exposure; (12) induced abortion; (13) genetic risk factors; and (14) prophylactic (preventive) mastectomy for women with high breast cancer risk.[7]

1. **Personal history of breast cancer.** Women with breast cancer have a three- to fourfold increased risk of developing a new cancer in the other breast.

Our personal history. Out of seventy women, nine had double mastectomies: two had both breasts removed at the same time, and seven had breasts removed at different intervals—one month, two months, six months, eight months, one year, two years, and six years.

2. **Previous Breast Biopsy.** Women whose previous breast biopsies indicated certain types of benign breast diseases (characterized as atypical hyperplasia) have a risk of breast cancer approximately five times that of the general population.

3. **Estrogen Replacement Therapy.** Some studies indicate that long-term use (ten years or more) of estrogen replacement therapy for relief of menopause symptoms may increase the risk of breast cancer. The American Cancer Society believes that the decision to use this hormone therapy after menopause should be made by the woman and her doctor after considering the possible positive and negative results of estrogen replacement therapy. Variables can include the risk for heart disease, breast cancer, and osteoporosis, and the severity of menopausal symptoms.

Discussion on the use of estrogen. The Orange County Register newspaper reported a new study in 1998: "Anti-osteoporosis drug rivals estrogen. Dr. Bess Dawson-Hughes, an osteoporosis researcher at Tufts University, is quoted as saying, 'Estrogen, in my view, would be the first line [of treatment], not only because it prevents bone loss, but it also prevents the progression of heart disease . . . and alleviates menopausal symptoms.' However, many women will not take estrogen because of its side effects and because of a modest increase in the risk of breast cancer, making alendronate (sold under the name of Fosamax) a good alternative."[8]

Dr. Susan Love, author of two books on breast cancer, is quoted in this same newspaper as saying, "We have to stop thinking about menopause as a disease that you need to take a pill to do something about. Menopause is a natural passage in life. . . . I am not against hormones . . . short-term." Dr. Love cautions that more research needs to be done before women take estrogen for twenty or thirty years, as taking estrogen does not necessarily protect a woman against osteoporosis, significantly reduce the risk of heart disease, or help women stay younger-looking.[9]

Our experiences with estrogen. Menopause presents difficult decisions for women. The decline in hormone production over a period of fifteen years produces many symptoms, including difficulty concentrating, poor memory, reduced stamina, itchy or dry skin, vaginal and urinary dryness, headaches, mood swings, declining sexual desire, hot flashes, loss of bone density, wrinkling, and other physical and emotional effects.

Jeannette (43/52) opposed estrogen replacement. "I had been given estrogen pills for hot flashes. Estrogen pills are dumb 'pumpkin' pills and should be thrown down the commode."

Personally, I have refused to take estrogen replacement therapy. I just can't imagine myself willfully taking anything that even remotely endangers my life again with the risk of cancer.

4. **Higher education or socioeconomic level.** There is increased risk of diagnosis of breast cancer for affluent women, but an increased mortality rate for those in poverty. Different lifestyle factors among women in upper socioeconomic classes may account for their added risk for breast cancer, when compared with those of less-educated and poorer women. However, specific factors giving an added risk for affluent women are not yet identified.

We did not discuss these topics. Higher education was required for those of us who were teachers, school administrators, and nurses. This does not preclude the possibility that the other women could have had higher education. It never occurred to me to ask, as cancer attacks both the educated and uneducated, the rich as well as the poor.

5. **Lifestyle Choices.** Researchers are finding that lifestyle choices may influence the risk of breast cancer. However, "experts from the United Kingdom and Republic of Ireland were less positive than respondents from other countries about the influence of stress, dietary fat, fiber and salt on disease. . . . Opinions differed widely about the influence of lifestyle on breast cancer and diabetes. . . . Experts were generally less likely to endorse lifestyle-disease links than those from other European countries."[10]

6. **Alcohol.** Some studies have shown that use of alcohol may be linked to increased risk of breast cancer. For those who drink alcoholic beverages, intake should be limited to one drink a day.

7. **Smoking.** While no studies have yet related cigarette smoking to breast cancer, it is known that smoking affects overall health and increases the risk for many other cancers, as well as heart disease.

8. **Overweight and high-fat diets.** Overweight, or obesity, has been implicated as a breast cancer risk in some studies, especially for women over fifty years of age. The exact mechanism and the level of risk remain subjects of intense research. In general, diets high in fat, especially the saturated fat in meat or dairy products, may increase breast cancer risk. However, studies to date are contradictory, and the level of increased risk remains to be defined.

9. **Exercise.** Exercise and cancer is a new area of research. A recent study indicated that strenuous exercise in youth may provide lifelong protection against some cancers, including breast cancer. Studies are underway to confirm these findings.

10. **Oral contraceptives.** Evidence regarding the role of oral contraceptives in increasing the risk of breast cancer still remains somewhat contradictory. However, a recent analysis using data from most of the large, well-designed published studies, found that women currently using oral contraceptives have a slightly greater risk of breast cancer than women not using oral contraceptives. Women who stopped using an oral contraceptive more than ten years ago do not appear to have any increased breast cancer risk. When considering using oral contraceptives, women should discuss their risk factors for breast cancer with their health-care team.

Our experiences with oral contraceptives. In my own experience, I was put on the birth-control pill in my early thirties because of endometriosis. This disorder results when tissue resembling the endometrium (the lining of the uterus) begins growing on the outside of the uterus and perhaps in other parts of the abdominal cavity.

Oral contraceptives combine estrogen and progestin. The side effects were (and are) weight gain, water retention, nausea, vaginal bleeding, and a slight increased risk of stroke. As many as 10 percent of women of reproductive age have endometriosis, and 30 to 40 percent of those diagnosed, experience notable pain, which I did. This disorder has been found to be a significant factor in female infertility. I was never blessed with pregnancy.

Dr. Duane Alexander advises, "Although it is generally agreed to be a common disorder, we really have no good data on its impact as a public health problem. We don't even have good information on its prevalence, in part because it is often misdiagnosed or under diagnosed, and because it varies widely according to the population that's under study."[11]

Endometriosis continues to baffle doctors and researchers. Although there is no cure for endometriosis, a variety of treatment options exists that include over-the-counter pain medication, hormonal therapy to stop ovulation for as long as possible (oral contraceptives), and surgery. Because of the severity of my endometriosis, I had the radical surgery, which involved hysterectomy, removal of all growths, and removal of ovaries. No cancer existed.

A few years later, when I needed a mastectomy, I asked my surgeon if there was a relationship between oral contraceptives and breast cancer. He said no and explained that while it was known that some cancers were estrogen dependent, researchers did not know which ones. I told him then that in the future, scientists would discover a connection between oral contraceptives and breast cancer, and they have.

Cancer specialists, researchers, and organizations describe risk factors in terms such as "only," "slightly," "small," "appears to," "no overall," "may," "usually," "no evidence," "probably." I believe they speak in these terms because they do not want to frighten people, and because their knowledge is limited. However, there are thousands of us walking around maimed from "only," "slightly," "small," "appears to," "no overall," "may," "usually," "no evidence," "probably."

Couching words has not minimized the results cancer inflicts upon our bodies. Vanessa (56/60) said, "While I was in the hospital, the nurses said they were getting a lot of women on the birth control pill with cancer, and that they personally were going to go off the pill. I am 'anti' hormone pills."

11. **Environmental exposure.** Additional factors that may be associated with increased breast cancer risk include pesticide and other chemical exposures in the environment. Research continues, as there is not yet data strong enough to establish a clear cause-effect relationship.

12. Induced abortion. A large recent study from Denmark has provided very strong data showing that induced abortions have no overall effect on the risk of breast cancer. There is no evidence of a direct relationship between breast cancer and spontaneous abortion in the majority of studies that have been published. Studies continue.

A note about this study. I believe women need to understand that this study by Dr. Mads Melbye of all women born in Denmark between the years of 1935 and 1978 (1.5 million) is highly controversial. Dr. Ron Gray, a Johns Hopkins professor of population dynamics, calls this the most solid study yet: "Solid because they had the information of breast cancer and abortion from registry records, so they didn't depend on the memory of respondents. So I think it's very reassuring that in the first trimester, there probably is no increased risk. What they did find was that in a very small proportion of women—about 3 percent, who had abortions later in pregnancy—there may have been some increased risk of breast cancer, and that really needs to be further researched."[12]

Those in opposition include Dr. Joel Brind, Ph.D., a professor of biology and endocrinology at Baruch College of the City University of New York: "…ten studies out of eleven on American women have shown increased risk, eight of them statistically significant on their own." Dr. Brind points to three major flaws in Melbye's study: (1) The inappropriate selection of computerized data from Danish birth, abortion and breast cancer registries; (2) invalid statistical adjustment of the raw data; (3) mischaracterization of their findings and of other published research in the field."[13]

Dr. J.C. Willke offers the following statistics:

> One woman in ten will develop breast cancer, and 25 percent will die. There are 1.6 million abortions each year in the United States: 56 percent are first abortions, 44 percent second or more. Over 800,000 women abort their first pregnancy each year. Of these, 10 percent or 80,000 would have developed breast cancer. But, because of their abortions, the number of cancer cases will increase to 120,000. Of these extra 40,000 cases, 25 percent, or 10,000 additional women will die of breast cancer every year.[14]

The editors of *New England Journal of Medicine Health News* conclude that the complex issue of whether abortion increases breast cancer is not easily resolved, and they ask, "…until more definitive evidence is available, how can you make sense of the evidence we do have?"[15]

Our group did not discuss abortion. The furthermost thing from my mind while interviewing was to discuss the death of a child by abortion. Our mothers had allowed us to live, and we were fighting for our very lives against cancer. We needed truthful information then, and we need truthful information today in our battle to live and defeat cancer. We need facts, not political manipulation of data.

Is there a link? Conflicting statistics and questionable evaluation of each research study leaves us with the quandary: Who can we trust? So many numbers are being tossed at us that conflict with one another. Benjamin Disraeli said there are three kinds of lies: "Lies, damned lies, and statistics."

I care about the women who have chosen to abort their babies. I care that they may have a higher risk for breast cancer. We all need to be concerned as 1.6 million abortions are performed each year in the United States. We are again presented the words "small risk," "no overall effect," and even a blanket "no risk." Do we not care that this "small risk" places thousands of young women in danger of cancer and possible death?

Remember that twenty-five years ago I questioned the relationship between oral contraceptives and breast cancer and was told that there was none, but today we know this relationship exists. It is not acceptable to me that today, some tell women there is no relationship between abortion and breast cancer. Do we wait another twenty-five years to say, "Oops! There is a relationship."?

We need valid, truthful, non-political, objective information about whether there is a connection between abortion and breast cancer. Until that is known, every women must be warned of cancer danger.

Getting more information. The Internet was not available to us in 1974–75. Today, anyone can have access to what is happening in cancer research worldwide. I encourage you to take advantage of this marvelous technology. If you don't have a computer, go to a library, local college, or ask a friend who has a computer to help you.

My perspective on abortion. As a Christian, I strongly oppose abortion-on-demand, and am particularly horrified, repelled, and anguished by the barbaric practice of late-term abortions. My heart breaks over the children and their children who are lost to us forever, created and loved by God. Perhaps such a child has been sent to us by God to bring us the cure for cancer and other such devastating diseases, but abortion got in the way of God's mercy.

13. **Genetic risk factors.** A personal or family history of breast cancer may make testing appropriate. Studies show that some breast cancer is hereditary and linked with mutations (or changes) of the BRCA1 and BRCA2 genes. Normally, these genes help to prevent cancer by making a protein that keeps cells from growing abnormally. However, if a person has inherited a mutated gene from either parent, this cancer-preventing protein is less effective, and the breasts are more susceptible to the development of cancer. About 50 to 60 percent of women with inherited BRCA1 mutations will develop breast cancer by the age of seventy. Women with these inherited mutations also have an increased risk for developing cancer of the ovary. Genetic testing can determine if a woman has inherited the mutated genes. It is done by analyzing DNA from a blood sample. If mutated genes are detected, the woman and her health team can take special care in watching for early signs of cancer or for growth of an additional tumor.

Additional findings. Two studies published in *The Journal of American Medical Association* "cast doubts on whether defective genes cause the early onset of breast cancer and how useful gene testing would be. The study from North Carolina found only three women among 211 breast cancer cases had a BRCA1 defect. The women were 20 to 74 years old and were selected without regard to whether they had a family history of the disease. In the Washington State study, only 12 women had a defective BRCA1 gene among 193 who developed breast cancer before age 35. Only 15 women had the trait among 208 who developed cancer before age 45 and also had a close relative with the disease."[16]

14. **Prophylactic (preventive) mastectomy for women with high breast cancer risk.** This is a surgical procedure infrequently chosen by some women at high risk for breast cancer. The purpose is to lessen their risk by removing one or both breasts at a time, when there is no known breast cancer. The reasons for using this type of surgery may include one, and usually even more, of the following risk factors: inheritance of mutated genes, previous cancer in one breast, strong family history (breast cancer in several close relatives), and biopsies showing lobular carcinoma in situ (LCIS) and/or atypical hyperplasia.

A controversial measure. This procedure is a controversial subject in the medical community. This operation removes nearly all of the breast tissue, but a small amount often remains. Although this operation reduces the risk of breast cancer, it cannot guarantee that a cancer will not develop in the small amount of breast tissue remaining after surgery. Second opinions are strongly recommended before any woman makes the decision to have this surgery. The American Cancer Society's board of directors has strongly stated that this type of preventive operation is warranted only if strong clinical and/or pathologic indications are evident.

A March 7, 1998, newspaper article entitled "Mixed results in study of preemptive surgery" was published in *The Orange County Register.* It reported another research study:

> Pre-emptive surgery to prevent breast and ovarian cancer in women who have high genetic risk should work based on computer projections, researchers said Friday. But while it should save lives, the surgery might not be worth it because the quality of life plummets, they said. Ever since BRCA1 and BRCA2 genes were identified, doctors have wondered whether it would be worth taking preventive action in women who have gene mutations known to lead to breast or ovarian cancer. Victor Grann and colleagues of Columbia University produced a computer model to see if preventive surgery could save the lives of women with a high genetic risk of cancer. They used input from the records of 14 million women and information from a panel of cancer specialists. Our analysis showed that women positive for the BRCA1 and BRCA2 gene mutations will survive longer if they have pro-

phylactic mastectomy (breast removal) and oophorectomy (removal of ovaries) than if they do not, they wrote in the *Journal of Clinical Oncology*.[17]

Our experiences with lobular carcinoma in situ (LCIS). Both Jennifer (27/27) and I (42/42) were diagnosed with lobular cancer, which develops in the milk-producing glands, but does not penetrate through the wall of the lobules. Women with LCIS are at increased risk of developing an invasive breast cancer in either breast over the long term and need to be monitored closely.

In 1974, Jennifer's surgeon said he'd seen only five women with lobular cancer that year and that only one of those women would not be having her second breast removed, opting instead to have it watched closely. The surgeon didn't think it was very wise or prudent to wait.

I told Jennifer that my surgeon never suggested I have the other breast removed, because he said there was only about a 10 percent chance that I would get cancer in the second breast. I suggested that we both get a second opinion.

When I phoned later to ask how she was, Jennifer indicated that both her husband and doctor did not want her to discuss breast removal, implants, or anything further with me. Twenty-five years later, I still have my other breast.

Summary of Risk Factors By American Cancer Society

Virtually all women will have one or more risk factors for breast cancer. However, most risks are at such a low level that they only partly explain the high frequency of the disease among women. To date, knowledge about risk factors has not translated into practical ways to prevent breast cancer. The best opportunity for reducing the death rate is through early detection.

Diagnosis of Breast Cancer: Mammography and Biopsy

Breast cancer develops over a period of years and can be present before any symptoms appear. The American Cancer Society offers these statistics: "When breast cancer is detected in a localized stage with no lymph node involvement, the five-year survival rate is 94 percent. If the cancer has spread to regional lymph nodes, the rate of survival drops to 73 percent."[18]

Mammography

Mammography, an x-ray technology, is the most widely used method for detecting breast abnormalities that are too small to see or feel. This technique produces a film image of a woman's breasts; the image is then reviewed by a radiologist. The radiation doses of the x-ray are very low and pose negligible risks for patients. The procedure takes approximately fifteen minutes. Compression of the breast is necessary to produce a good mammogram and may cause some momentary discomfort.

The radiologist will be looking for abnormalities that can range from findings that are clearly cancerous in appearance, to tiny calcium deposits (microcalcification), which are usually benign. It may become necessary to return and have the mammogram repeated. Ultrasound scans (an imaging method using sound waves) may also be ordered. A few studies have shown that fear of breast cancer keeps some high-risk women from obtaining mammograms, particularly those with less formal education.

Our experiences with mammography. Except for more sophisticated machines today, the procedure is the same as it was for those of us who had the testing several years ago, and it is nothing to fear. The most difficult part is waiting to hear the results, and this can cause unexpected anxiety. I turn to prayer.

When results are unclear, a woman is called back for another mammogram. This happened to me in 1997, and the second mammogram confirmed an area of microcalcifications. These are tiny calcium deposits within the breast, singly or in clusters. This sign of change may be monitored by additional, periodic mammograms, or by immediate or delayed biopsy. Calcium deposits may be caused by cancer or by aging and are very common.

My internist admitted that doctors often are overly concerned about a patient who has already had one breast removed. A biopsy was recommended, and my family insisted that I do so. The biopsy was performed on June 19, 1997, and was benign.

Biopsy

When suspicious areas are found through mammography, a biopsy (tissue sample) is the only way to tell if the abnormality is cancerous. The biopsy is then examined under a microscope. There are several types of biopsies, including fine-needle aspiration biopsy, core biopsy, and surgical biopsy. The American Cancer Society offers the following information concerning five biopsy options:[19]

1. **Fine-Needle Aspiration Biopsy (FNAB).** This procedure uses a thin needle, about the size of a needle used for blood tests or for immunizations. Stereotactic biopsy uses a computer-guided x-ray needle to take a sample of the suspicious area discovered on a mammogram, but it is too small to be felt. This procedure is often used to biopsy calcifications (calcium deposits). Applying suction to the needle (aspiration) during FNAB may yield fluid. Clear fluid usually indicates a benign cyst, while bloody or cloudy fluid may be present in benign cysts or cancers. In some cases, a clear answer is not obtained by FNAB, and another type of biopsy is needed.

Additional information about FNAB. The Memorial Sloan-Kettering Cancer Center indicates,

> Breast-imaging specialists in the Department of Radiology are now refining and demonstrating the benefit of stereotactic needle biopsy. . . . For many women, stereotactic needle biopsy can spare them a more uncomfortable and expensive surgical biopsy. It can also allow them to start their treatment sooner. . . . According to radiologist Dr. Laura Liberman, stereotactic needle biopsy is still vastly underutilized in the United States. Because of its benefits to women and the cost savings, it should be used more widely, she said. 'If you find a woman's cancer early, you can save her life.'[20]

My personal experience with fine-needle aspiration biopsy and surgical biopsy in 1997. My surgeon explained the stereotactic needle biopsy option but said that there could be no guarantee with this procedure, as the needle would be touching only a portion of the area in question and may miss the cancer. He gave me three options: (1) wait and monitor with another mammogram in three months; (2) use the stereotactic needle biopsy; or (3) have a surgical biopsy, which would completely remove the area in question. I chose this third option, as my family was also concerned, and it is the surest protection known today.

The surgery is nothing to fear. I entered the hospital as an outpatient. The area designated for surgery was marked with needles so fine that I did not even feel them being placed. I was given anesthesia, and the surgery took less than an hour. I was able to go home approximately an hour afterward, but because of the anesthesia, I did not drive myself. I found very little discomfort while healing. There is a degree of bruising that caused discoloration of my breast, but that disappeared within several days.

I later discovered a hard nodule under the incision, and the surgeon felt quite confident that it was only dead tissue. Because I wanted to make sure, he arranged for me to have a fine-needle aspiration on February 11, 1998.

As an assistant prepared me for the procedure, I asked if she were examining her own breasts, and she said, "No, I'm only in my thirties."

As I told her of the importance of doing so, the radiologist reentered the room and said, "I am glad you are talking to her. I have been trying to get her to do BSE for a long time."

I was saddened that here was a young woman working in the medical field and being encouraged by her radiologist but still not taking BSE seriously.

Do not fear a fine-needle aspiration. The radiologist injects a small amount of anesthetic with a tiny needle into the skin over the lump. Then, using a needle, the size used to draw blood, he or she punctures the lump several times (usually fewer than six times) and makes smears on slides of the material obtained.

My radiologist gives a fact sheet that cautions,

It is important for you to understand that this procedure is not foolproof. It does not always provide a definitive diagnosis, and sometimes I do not even get sufficient material to evaluate at all (in which case you are invited for a free return engagement should you want to try again). Remember also that finding only benign cells is not a guarantee that something worse was not present but not sampled.

The site of the punctures may ache afterward, like a bruise, and indeed may be bruised. Local ice in the first twenty-four hours will help reduce swelling and pain. If discomfort persists, switch to local, warm compresses after the first day. If the puncture site is dry, you can bathe or shower two hours after the procedure.

I had no bruising and very little discomfort. The radiologist then promised "the most bizarre Band-Aid I have available, and you're on your way." I had envisioned a huge dressing, because of the word *bizarre*. Oh, how I laughed when he placed a tiny comic-strip character Band-Aid on my breast. I loved his ability to lighten up a situation that brings anxiety to women. His humor carried me through the twenty-four hours I spent waiting for the results to be conveyed to my surgeon.

The aspiration confirmed my surgeon's view of fat necrosis, which is common. The larger the breast (which describes me), the more likelihood there is that fat necrosis will develop. Fat necrosis is dead fat, and results because the blood supply to fat is always poor, and many events around the time of surgery can interfere with blood supply, such as too much pressure being used on an area.

The aspiration was benign. I mused aloud to the radiologist that I could not possibly have any credibility in writing this book if I had refused to have the biopsy, and now the aspiration.

He said, "Good, you not only talk the talk, you walk the walk."

2. **Core biopsy.** This procedure uses a larger needle than in FNAB. It removes a small cylinder of tissue and is done with local anesthesia in the doctor's office.

3. **Nipple discharge procedure.** If there is a nipple discharge, some of the fluid may be collected and then examined under a microscope to determine if any cancer cells are present. A special x-ray may also be performed after injecting x-ray contrast material into the duct or ducts from which the spontaneous discharge is coming.

4. **Surgical biopsy.** This procedure involves the removal of all, or a portion, of the lump for microscopic analysis.

Two-step biopsy. Today, most health professionals prefer a two-step biopsy. In this method, the biopsy usually can be done in the doctor's office or hospital outpatient department under a nongeneral anesthesia with intravenous sedation or local anesthesia with the woman being awake during the procedure. If the diagnosis is cancer, there is time to learn about it, discuss all treatment options with the cancer care-team, friends, and family. The short delay until treatment does no harm. Of course, a diagnosis made by needle biopsy counts as the first step of a two-step procedure.

Today's biopsy advantages. In previous years, the only choice a woman had was a one-step biopsy. With this approach, she was given general anesthesia and was asleep during the entire process. A biopsy was performed, and the tissue sample was frozen. The frozen sample was examined in the pathology laboratory under a microscope. If cancer cells were present, the surgeon immediately proceeded with treatment, such as mastectomy, which the patient had previously approved. The patient did not know until she woke up whether the lump had been cancerous and whether surgery had been performed. Today, this approach is rarely recommended.

Our biopsy options in 1974–1975. We were given both options of either a two-step biopsy or a one-step biopsy. Some chose the two-step biopsy. I chose the one-step biopsy because I had done a lot of research before the surgery and knew much of what to expect. My doctor also explained the effects of anesthesia being administered twice, and I did not want to subject my body to that additional stress.

5. **Estrogen/progesterone receptors.** Receptors are part of the molecular structure of a cell, functioning as a "welcome mat" for certain substances that circulate in the blood. Certain tumor cells have hormone receptors, which will recognize estrogen and progesterone. These two substances play an important role in the development, treatment, and prognosis of certain tumors. An important step in evaluating a person with early breast cancer is to test for the presence of these receptors. This is done on a portion of the cancerous tissue to be removed at the time of biopsy or initial surgical treatment. Knowledge about your receptors provides important information relating to future hormone therapy which can affect the outlook, or prognosis, of a woman's breast cancer.

Life Is Sacred to Me

Fear, denial, and procrastination can keep us from saving our lives. In 1974, a woman had given me the name of her friend—Fay—and had asked me to phone and encourage Fay, who needed surgery for breast cancer. Fay angrily said she did not want counseling, refused a mastectomy, and was resentful that her friend had given me her name and phone number. This loving friend later told me that Fay's choice resulted in death.

Jackie, a nurse, shared, "Women are totally frightened and think more of death. They feel loss of control over the situation, anger at the possible loss of sexuality as breasts denote womanhood, and feel less complete. They feel helpless and hopeless."

I believe that life is sacred and to be held in reverence, not viewed as something helpless and hopeless. "If [we] come across an insect which has fallen into a puddle, [we] stop a moment in order to hold out a leaf or a stalk on which it can save itself."[21] We women hold out this book to you as our leaf to encourage you to make choices that will help save your life. Please reject the idea of hopelessness, and instead, affirm that life is hope.

> *"Thou art he that took me out of the womb;*
> *thou didst make me hope*
> *when I was upon my mother's breasts."*
> —*Psalm 22:9*

"Reputation is what men and women think of us; character is what God and angels know of us."

—THOMAS PAINE
American political philosopher
(1737–1809)

3

SELECTING
THE RIGHT DOCTORS

"The best portion of a good man's life is his little,
nameless, unremembered acts of kindness and love."
—*William Wordsworth*
English poet (1770–1850)

WE HAVE JUST READ ABOUT STATISTICS, risk factors, and guidelines that exist for cancer patients. The importance of selecting a family doctor in whom we have confidence and trust cannot be overstated.

Acceptance and adjustment to cancer is greatly affected by the nature of the patient-doctor relationship. "Clear and open communication, expression of appropriate emotion, and collaborative planning and problem-solving enhance adjustment and improve outcome. Conversely, influences that isolate breast cancer patients from others or undermine support can have adverse medical and psychological consequences."[1]

Dr. Craig M. Walker, medical director of the Cardiovascular Institute of the South, suggests,

> Your best chance of obtaining the proper treatment for this or any condition requiring the care of a specialist would continue to lie with your selection of the right doctor. This means

choosing a (doctor) with the right training, professional certification, and ready access to the opinions of a broad range of
equally qualified colleagues in all the appropriate surgical and
nonsurgical subspecialties. . . . Guidelines or no guidelines, the
selection and conduct of your treatment is going to rest, ultimately, on one physician's best judgment. You want that
judgment to be as informed and unbiased as possible. And if
your insurance company doesn't require a second opinion,
. . . obtain one anyway. Second opinions are good medical practice, and no responsible physician would consider it an affront
to his or her judgment if you seek one.[2]

How Can We Research Physicians?

- Patients can call state medical licensing boards to check
  physicians' licenses. How much information is available
  varies.
- Some states post physician license information on the Internet. Administrators in Medicine runs a free "Docfinder"
  site that links to about a dozen states. The address is
  http://docboard.madriver.com. The American Board of
  Medical Specialties also can provide some information on a
  physician's board certification at www.certifieddoctor.org.
- The only public comprehensive list of doctor discipline,
  which includes fifty States' records of Medicare and Drug
  Enforcement Administration sanctions, is Public Citizen's
  "16,638 Questionable Doctors." The group is not posting
  the information on the Internet and will charge consumers
  for each book of local information. To request information, call (202) 588-7780.
- The American Medical Association recommends its
  "Physician Select" Internet site at www.ama-assn.org/aps/
  amahg.htm. It tells whether a doctor is an AMA member,
  where he or she went to school, his or her board certification, and some other details, but doesn't discuss discipline.
- Experts suggest asking friends, other doctors, hospitals and
  local medical societies for physician recommendations.
  Ask if a doctor has admitting privileges to a convenient
  hospital.[3]

How Do We Protect Ourselves When Selecting Doctors?

Solid information about the quality of U.S. medicine is still lacking today. Ron Police, executive director of the health consumer group Families USA, said, "For the overwhelming majority of Americans, good useful, practical information is not at their fingertips."[4] Experts caution that it could be years before data currently being collected can help people choose doctors.

There is future hope, in that many experts are trying to ascertain which treatments work best and are the most cost effective. They are also developing methods to provide better information for the patients for comparing the quality of health plans, hospitals, and doctors. "This is a field that's just exploding right now," said David Shulkin, chief medical officer and quality officer at the University of Pennsylvania Health System.[5] Thus the competition between HMOs for patients is projected to benefit the consumer by forcing HMOs to compete on the basis of quality of care.

What Do We Look for in Choosing a Doctor?

In 1974–1975, we were able to have doctors who spent time with each patient and thus built a precious doctor-patient relationship. But with today's managed care, doctors usually schedule patients every fifteen minutes, which for patients, often results in confusion, anger, and a lack of trust.

This strained relationship is being recognized as destructive, and an encouraging research is being conducted by the University of California at Irvine (UCI) with the intent of teaching physicians how to have a better bedside manner. This study is seeking answers to "whether doctors can change their behavior, if the changes increase patient satisfaction, and whether UCI should extend communication training to all its physicians and residents."[6] Based on this training being conducted by the Bayer Institute of Health Care Communication, a patient should look for the following indicators when choosing a doctor: a doctor who

- maintains eye contact and expresses warmth.
- expresses interest in you as well as in your illness.

- begins by asking an open-ended question and doesn't interupt your opening statement.
- finds out all your complaints and negotiates an agenda about what to address now and what to address during a later visit.
- summarizes your feelings to make sure they're correct. Asks if you understand his or her instructions and viewpoints.
- encourages you to ask questions.[7]

This training would please Nurse Clara (59/71), who pleaded the importance of a good bedside manner: "There is a great need for kindness, there is a great need for touching."

Nurse Jackie also would applaud. "Doctors do not meet the emotional needs of women. Nurses meet the total needs of the patient. Doctors meet only the physical need and are not tuned into the total person."

Today, my cousin Rita, an experienced nurse, expresses additional concerns:

> Nurses are not wanting to face the fact that a person will die; they just want to help cure. Surgeons think surgery is the answer; they do it and then walk away. Doctors don't always answer your questions even when you ask them. Perhaps it is the fact of cancer, a lot to be absorbed in itself. Twenty-five years ago, doctors were not taught what they need to know. They looked at people with diseases, but not as a whole person. Tell all women to make a list of questions before they go to the doctors. Write them down, and take the list with you so you won't forget what to ask. Young women are not just fearful, I think they are in denial: 'This can't happen to me.'

How Did I Choose My Internist?

My husband and I lost our beloved young internist, who suddenly died in November 1997, and I am still grieving his death. We sought someone with his qualities and have been blessed to find, in his office, another splendid internist whose compassionate heart and bedside manner guide her competent skills, and who agrees with our medical philosophy of not taking heroic measures in terminal cases. She is a gem, as are the colleagues she refers us to outside her expertise. We are delighted with the quality of doctors used by our HMO, Secure Horizons.

When Should We Seek a Second Opinion?

We must not hesitate to ask questions. Many doctors advise patients to walk away from any doctor who takes a question as a personal affront or tells us not to worry because he or she will take care of it.

Ethel (41/47)

warned us to be sure to see more than one doctor. "My doctor told me not to worry about statistics. He said I was cured after a year. I didn't believe him." (The surgeon who did my biopsy in 1997 said the doctors he knows no longer tell patients they are permanently cured, as cancer is a lifetime disease and women should remain hopefully vigilant.)

Margaret (48/49)

asked me to be sure to tell you to get more than one doctor's opinion before agreeing to the mastectomy. She worried that she would hurt her doctor's feelings if she had sought a second opinion, but she doesn't want us to make the same mistake. "If I had done it, cancer would not have gone as far as it did."

Nurse Clara (59/71)

agreed: "I would advise women to have more than one surgeon examine the lump. Any doctor who does not want to talk to you should have a nurse in his office that is able to talk to you."

I firmly agree that a second opinion should always be sought in life-threatening situations, should time permit. Ethel, Margaret, and Clara would find that getting a second opinion today under HMOs managed care is more complicated and difficult than what we experienced without HMOs.

Even though today many doctors, patients, and advocates are insisting upon the importance and urgency of second opinions from doctors outside of the same managed-care plan, there is not agreement, as various bills begin to move through the legislature.

Mark Sektnan, a lobbyist for the California Association of Health Plans, said the industry insisted on the more limited language of allowing a second opinion only from a doctor within the same managed-care plan. "We wanted to maintain some kind of control over second opinions. You don't want people to go doctor shopping."[8]

So what is the tentative legislation agreement concerning patient rights to seek a second opinion? Assembly Bill 341:

- The patient questions the reasonableness or necessity of recommended surgical procedure.
- The patient questions a diagnosis or plan of care for a condition that threatens the loss of life, loss of limb, loss of bodily function or substantial impairment of that function.
- The patient requests an additional diagnosis when clinical indications are not clear or are complex and confusing; a diagnosis is in doubt because of conflicting test results; or the doctor is unable to diagnose the condition.
- The treatment plan in progress is not improving the patient's medical condition.
- The patient has serious concerns about the diagnosis or plan of care and has attempted to follow the plan and consulted his or her original physician.[9]

The importance of having a second opinion has remained constant over the years. It is ironic that we must now apply to the Legislature to pass laws allowing procedures we had in the first place in 1974–1975 without HMOs managed care. Does anyone doubt the wisdom and necessity of asking questions of the current health-care system in the United States?

How We Chose Our Doctors

Surgeons were chosen primarily on the recommendations of a trusted family doctor, nursing staffs, and friends who'd had cancer surgery. The ideal doctor was described not only as being knowledgeable, well trained, up-to-date, and competent, but also as having a caring bedside manner. Vivid memories surfaced during the interviews. No woman hesitated in expressing strong emotions and opinions concerning how their doctors treated them as cancer patients.

Our Competent Doctors with a Bedside Manner

Bernice (43/44):

"I had known my family doctor for ten years, and I had faith in him that he would not send me to a surgeon who was going to harm me. My surgeon's attitude gave me confidence more than anything, because I didn't know what his credentials were. He is confident, honest with me, never beats around the bush, and has answered all my questions. Anything he doesn't tell me is not because he is holding things back. He knows so much, and sometimes you just forget to tell things, overlooking details that are just minor to you but to others are important. I do that. I have talked to three women that have had him and think he is great."

Sarah (44/44):

"I still feel the surgeon is an excellent surgeon. He did the best he could. He did the best in his power and I would highly recommend him. The nurses just love him. One nurse told me not to worry about when he would be around because all the nurses flock around when they know he will be in the building."

Marie (42/42):

Bernice, Sarah, and I had never met prior to the interviews, but we had the same surgeon, and I wholeheartedly agree with their appraisal of him. My husband and I trusted our family doctor completely, so when he gave us a list of three surgeons to consider, I began to interview all three. I also phoned the head nurses at three hospitals to ask who the nursing staff would recommend. I knew they would say they could not give such information, but each head nurse said they would be willing to respond if I gave them a surgeon's name.

My final choice of a surgeon hinged on the facts that he had been recommended by my family doctor and the head nurse at the hospital where he practiced; he was knowledgeable, honest, patient, kind, and self-confident; and the hospital was close to our home, which would help my husband cope. As Bernice stated, our surgeon's attitude also gave me confidence.

Alice (39/47):

"The doctor didn't tell me anything. When I was a kid, I had to stay around a person having cancer, to help out, so cancer was a scary word. Cancer is not a scary word today because there is so much help if they get there in time and not let it go like me. It was like being ignorant. I didn't know anything then. After the mastectomy, my doctor helped me to adjust. He just had that bedside manner."

Donna (41/42):

"My family doctor was on vacation, and when he came back, I felt better. The surgeon talked to my husband and me for about an hour-and-a-half. I had never met him before. He spoke of what would happen if it were malignant. He gave quotes from doctors from New York and other famous doctors about the types of mastectomy. I really wasn't listening. I thought, *What a nice man to come in and do this.* I know my husband was listening more than I was. I was half listening and half thinking, *I hope this isn't going to be true.*"

Glenda (55/55):

"My daughter is a cardiopulmonary therapist and wanted me to ask the nursing staff who they felt were the most highly qualified surgeons because their patients got well faster than others did, and they were the talk of the hospital of how beautifully they performed. The surgeon I chose gave me such an extensive examination. He did explain the options of surgery because it depended very much on the location of the thing. The medical profession came to the conclusion six months ago that a radical mastectomy was not any more effective, unless cancer had progressed to the point of lymph node involvement. He discussed the new chemotherapy, as they had stopped using cobalt six months ago. He said that Betty Ford had a radical because she was with the older type doctors, and Happy Rockefeller had a newer method. I just felt he knew. Maybe that is what I wanted to hear."

Esther (44/57):

"The surgeon was a friend of my doctor. When I was in the hospital with pain, I felt better hearing his footsteps coming down the hall. He had kindness, always came in with a whistle, always cheerful. He just made me feel better."

Kent, husband of Beth (40/51), who had died before our interview:

"My wife had a surgeon who was a kind, understanding, sensitive man. Her oncologist is a serious, bright young man. You will love him."

Our Competent Doctors with No Bedside Manner

Kitty (29/31):

"My surgeon was super cold, not a warm man. He was never warm but pretty honest in answering my questions. Most doctors would not take me because I was on Laetrile, which is illegal in the United States. I at last found a doctor through my nurse friend who at least checked my blood. Then I got a cancer doctor whom I like very much. He is not terribly warm, but I have confidence in him."

Martha (78/79):

"My surgeon was very gruff and sharp speaking, even though he was a good surgeon."

Olivia (45/54):

"My surgeon is a man of few words. I have great faith in his ability, but he had no bedside manner. Yet I would go back to him because I think he is a marvelous surgeon. He is straight. I was given no alternative: if it was malignant, I would be given a radical mastectomy."

Grace (46/57):

"I would think that one chooses a doctor on the basis of his skill. My surgeon was a very sober man. I never was able to get a smile out of him. It was not possible to get much interaction with him. He was a grim man, and I felt sorry for him. His assistant was a great, young, outgoing, fun doctor. Doctors need to be more humane and more concerned with their patients. They need to train more doctors, open more medical schools. Good heaven! When people have to stand in line for days to see a doctor, and then you are rushed in and out, we need more doctors and we need better care."

All Our Doctors Are Subject to Human Error

Jennifer (27/27):

"My doctor said he would bet his life that the lump was not malignant, just a fibroma. He said, 'I have been right and have only missed two in all my practice.' I told him, 'That was not a clogged duct, I know my breast better than you do.' I should have pushed it more. I felt sort of dumb. Even my husband said if the doctor said it is insignificant, don't worry about it. My case is different because it fooled everybody. Two prominent doctors in the area missed it, a surgeon and an OB. Nobody thought it was cancer."

Robin (60/62):

"Doctors should not tell patients they are pretty sure it is not cancer, as it may be. Doctors should tell patients about prosthesis. My two doctors had never seen one. They should know, even though they are very busy."

Vanessa (56/60):

"As a widow, my doctor started me on premerin, a hormone. He said it might cause breast cancer. I said I didn't want anything that would endanger my life, as my son's father was dead. When I needed a D&C, I asked why the first doctor had kept me on hormone pills if doctors don't know enough about the side effects of premerin. Doctors sure stick together, but the second doctor seemed to be honest when he said that the Mayo Clinic tests made them think that four months on premerin should not hurt me."

Margaret (48/49):

"I'm from Belgium, and they don't go to a doctor until they are half dead. I knew nothing about mastectomies. My doctor wanted to explain, but I said I didn't want to know. I didn't want him to go into details. I just told him to do what you have to do. You have five different doctors, you get five different opinions. Another thing I've learned is that doctors are all prima donnas. They all think they are right."

Della (47/52):

"As a registered nurse, I have known a great many surgeons and chose mine because he is humane, rigid, and up-to-date. He is well disciplined himself, and I could depend upon him to make all the right decisions. My doctor kept assuring me that it was benign. I had known him for so many years and had great faith. He is still my doctor. He is a friend, and I know he does not like to do mastectomies, as he told me that is one surgery he does not like to do.

"He was disturbed that he had let it go that long, because even when I went into the hospital, he had written on the report that there was only 10 percent chance of it being malignant. I think he really wanted to believe that. It was negligence, and I wasn't happy about it, but being a nurse I realize that these things happen. I guess I accept the fallacies of doctors more than most people, because I see it every day. I don't have total faith in the medical profession. There is a great difference of opinion, even among radiologists. Each one has a different theory on what should be done."

Andrea (39/43):

"My husband is a pediatrician. Doctor's wives get better care as far as the pathology report. They don't get better care otherwise. Everybody should get the same kind of scrupulous study, and there should be a uniform type of study. I don't know how the average individual makes sure this is done. You have to trust the Pathology Department, have faith they are functioning properly, because nine times out of ten, they probably are. Hopefully, within the next five years, there won't be many women dying from it, because they will find these lumps and have the courage to get themselves to the doctor.

"First and foremost, the doctors should not put them off. My husband is a doctor. My father was a doctor. I was raised in a medical family, but I have a thing about doctors. I don't like very many of them. They have set themselves up as little tin gods who are determined to decide what is right for us. The first person that has to be educated is the doctor. I feel very strongly about this. They probably are being educated today, one way or another, either from their patients or hopefully in school."

Nurse Clara (59/71)

pleads for kindness and understanding on the part of doctors: "I am seventy-one and had a Halsted radical mastectomy at the age of fifty-nine. I had a surgeon who was just a cold-blooded fish, whose own office staff said he does a good surgical job, but he doesn't want to talk to his patients. He is that kind of man, a good surgeon and a good mechanic. They charitably say he just does not have a bedside manner.

"As a nurse, I know the bedside manner is terribly important in a mastectomy. When a woman loses her breast or is told she will lose her breast and it is malignant, she requires some form of professional understanding and explanation of it that will soften the cold facts of it.

"You are lost—at least I was—because the worst people in the world are medical people for any kind of patient-doctor relationship. Doctors are not good patients themselves. But I had been trained for years in kindness and understanding and trying to put myself in the place of the patient, and I was a good nurse. I didn't get any of that, I didn't even get a doctor who came around my bed and put his hand on me and say, 'I'm sorry it had to be, but you are going to be all right, because I know we got everything.'

"In a female, when this has happened and she has lost part of what is her actual womanhood, there is a great need for kindness; there is a great need for touching. I'm a great believer in just that much [she lightly touched my arm], but my surgeon never did, and he never did explain.

"I have been in the medical profession for forty-five years, and I size doctors up rather coldly and perhaps unmercifully. If you know a nurse, ask her about a doctor. Or call the county medical if you are new in the area. They will give you three names. I would shop. Are they a good surgeon, well trained, good mechanic, personality? You can tell when a person is a good human being. I had a surgeon who just didn't give a darn except that his surgery was right."

> *"Be kind and merciful. Let no one ever come*
> *to you without coming away better and happier.*
> *Be the living expression of God's kindness:*
> *kindness in your face, kindness in your eyes,*
> *kindness in your warm greeting . . . to all who*
> *suffer and are lonely, give always a happy smile.*
> *Give them not only your care, but also your heart."*
> —Mother Teresa
> *Catholic Nun, Nobel Peace Prize (1910–1997)*

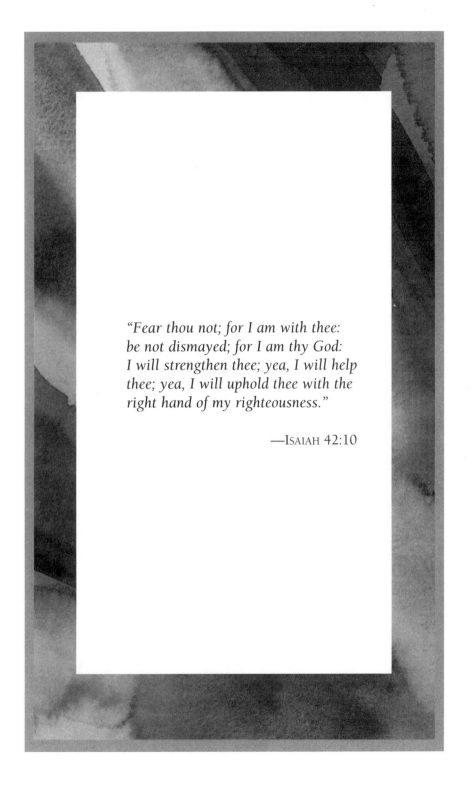

"Fear thou not; for I am with thee:
be not dismayed; for I am thy God:
I will strengthen thee; yea, I will help
thee; yea, I will uphold thee with the
right hand of my righteousness."

—Isaiah 42:10

4

SURGERY AND TREATMENT

"Courage is resistance to fear,
mastery of fear, not absence of fear."
—*Mark Twain*
American humorist (1835–1910)

TIME SEEMS SUSPENDED WHILE WAITING for the results of mammo-grams and biopsies. Anxiety results in frustration over delayed radiologist and pathology reports. We seek instant feedback as we are on an emotional seesaw that denies us peace. *Let it not be cancer* is our prayer.

When the report is benign, exhilaration overtakes us. When told we have breast cancer, our initial reactions range from hys-terical denial to quiet acceptance. We are in a state of numbing shock, often followed by tears, denial, anger, apprehension, and depression. We fear the possibility of dying and leaving loved ones who need us. In dazed disbelief and semi-awareness, we hear our doctors explain the stages of breast cancer, surgery options, and decisions that must be made.

Identifying the Stages of Invasive Breast Cancer

- *Stage I:* The tumor is 2.0 cm (about 3/4-inch) or less in diam-eter with no spread to the underarm (axillary) lymph nodes.

- *Stage II:* The tumor is over 2.0 cm (3/4-inch in diameter), and/or has spread to the underarm (axillary) lymph nodes which remain movable.
- *Stage III:* The breast cancer is more advanced with the tumor larger than 5.0 cm (2 inches) in diameter and/or involving lymph nodes under the arm, which are attached to one another or adjacent tissues.
- *Stage IV:* Regardless of the size of the tumor in the breast, the definition of Stage IV means that the cancer has already spread to distant organs or to lymph nodes in the neck above the collar bone (supraclavicular lymph nodes).[1]

Identifying the Types of Breast Cancer Surgery

1. *Lumpectomy* involves the removal of only the lump and a rim of normal tissue. Some of the underarm lymph nodes may be removed to see if the cancer has spread.
2. *Partial or segmental mastectomy or quadrantectomy* removes up to one-quarter or more of the breast, depending on the findings. Axillary lymph nodes under the arm also may be removed.
3. *Simple or total mastectomy* involves the removal of the entire breast.
4. *Modified radical mastectomy* involves the removal of the entire breast and axillary lymph nodes.
5. *Radical mastectomy* is the very extensive removal of the entire breast, axillary lymph nodes, and the chest wall muscles under the breast. This surgery was once very common, but because of its disfigurement and side effects, is now rarely done.[2]

What Are Our Chances for Survival?

Scientifically, our survival may be determined by several factors, including: (1) size of the tumor; (2) tumor's hormone sensitivity that is related to estrogen or progesterone receptors; and (3) type and maturity of the tumor cells, and how far the cancer has spread (metastasis).

No doctor can say specifically how an individual will respond to cancer and treatment, since we are unique unto ourselves physically and emotionally. Positives in our favor include general good health, family support, belief in ourselves, and our deep faith in God.

What Do Statistics Tell Us about Survival?

Ina Pilgrim in her book, *The Topic of Cancer,* informs us: "Survival in breast cancer treated by radical mastectomy is related to the size of the tumor when it is removed. If the tumor is less than 2 cm (3/4 of an inch) in diameter, then five-year survival is about 76 percent; if it is 2 to 5 cm (3/4 to 2 inches) in diameter, the five-year survival is 55 percent; and if the tumor is 5 to 10 cm (2 to 4 inches) in diameter, then the five-year survival is about 25 percent. . . . In untreated breast cancer, 85 percent of the women diagnosed as having it will live for a year; 50 percent will live for two-and-a-half years, and 20 percent will live past five years (the usual criterion for the cure of the disease)."[3]

Statistical limitations. One of the most difficult things that a person with cancer has to deal with is the fact that one is never sure whether the operation has actually cured the disease or not. Two women may have breast cancers that appear the same in size and type. They may undergo surgery by the same surgeon, and yet one dies two years later while the other survives forty years to die from complications resulting from a broken hip, not from cancer.

We Chose to Fight for Our Lives, and Fight We Did!

When unwelcome fear accompanied us into the surgery room, we also took courage with us. We relied on the skill of our surgeons and their hospital staffs. Some of us put our faith and trust in God, knowing that He would never leave us alone in the midst of our struggles. Our dreams were of life and recovery and of continued loving relationships with family and friends. Awaking from surgery, we were grateful to be alive.

Jennifer (27/27): "I want implants."

"The biopsy report showed that it was a cancerous lump. I had to tell my husband, and you always wonder how far it has gone; has it gotten into my lymph nodes? My husband said, 'I don't believe it, they told us it wasn't.' He sat there and tried to talk me out of it. He kept saying, 'They took a biopsy, this can't be, they told us it wasn't.' I said, 'Don't try to talk me out of it.'

"The doctor drew pictures about lumpectomy, modified radical, and radical mastectomies prior to the surgery. He didn't think the lumpectomy would make sure. As it turned out, I had two lumps that he had missed. In the radical, they take out the pectoral muscles, a group of muscles that are connected with your nodes. He was pretty specific. He said that there had been a study done in England that showed that after ten years, those who only had lumpectomy had a higher mortality rate than those with a modified radical. He dismissed the Halsted radical [originating in 1889] by saying he didn't think it was being done in California anymore as the surgeons feel it is far too drastic. I didn't know anything about mastectomy before this.

"In the hospital, I didn't think of anything. I noticed the fern in my room and had to call my girlfriend to thank her for it. I experienced numbness after surgery more than anything. [The doctor] had warned me that I would be numb, but you never really know until it happens.

"I was twenty-seven, and all the nurses were young, like under thirty. I had one nurse who didn't come back for two days, and I asked her why. She said, 'I don't know how you can do it and be so happy.' I asked her if she had been sick, and she said no. Then I realized that it was me that was affecting her. Then I realized that I was affecting all these girls on the staff. They could identify with me as a woman. It wasn't as if I had an operation on my foot. They all went home and asked their husbands, 'What would you do if this happened to me?' Their husbands all said they would just be glad that they were alive and said all the things that girls like to hear.

"Radiation was not discussed until after the pathology report. The doctor said if it wasn't in the lymph nodes, it had not gotten any place else. I had lobular cancer. There is a difference of opinion of whether it occurs in the second breast: some think

20 percent chance and others 100 percent. My doctor thinks about 80 percent of the time, but he would not commit himself. It won't metastasize there, but you have a predisposition toward it, and the other breast will get it within five to ten years. He said it is a low-grade cancer, but I don't want you to think it is not cancer, as it is cancer. He said it would be my decision, but he would strongly recommend that my other breast come off. He said he has had only five women with lobular cancer this year, and only one of them won't have the second breast removed, but wants it watched. He didn't think that was very wise or prudent to do. They said that lobular cancer does not show up on x-rays.

"I'm going to have the other breast removed in January. I talked to another doctor who was a plastic surgeon. He thought it was more of a 20 percent chance that the other breast would get cancer. My question was, Should I have the lymph nodes removed or just have the breast tissues scooped out? He said, just scooped. They will leave the skin, scrape the ribs like they did over here, and put in a silicone implant. I did not seek the advice of another surgeon as he wanted copies of the first surgery, mammography, etc. It was the holidays, so my husband and I said the heck with it."

[I later phoned Jennifer. She had her second breast removed two weeks after the above interview. There was no sign of cancer but active cells. She had implants at the same time, but said her doctor did not want her to show me the implants. However, she would ask him and call me. Jennifer never did phone.]

Kitty (29/31): "I feared metastasis."

"I was separated from my first husband and baby-sat ten children, plus my two, so a friend had to take over for me while I went into the hospital. My family was in northern California, and I didn't tell them until it was over, because if it wasn't malignant, I did not want to worry them. Naturally they were very upset when I did tell them. One of my friends was super. I knew that if I awoke to find a small bandage I was all right, but if not, it was cancer. So she waited around several hours to tell me, as the doctor did not tell me.

"The doctor explained that if cancer came back, it would go to the lungs, liver, or bone. They could use chemotherapy, but that would all be delaying tactics and not a guaranteed cure. If it came back into the bone and was isolated, it might be treatable with radiation. If it went to the liver or lungs, they could not radiate these tissue areas, and could only use chemotherapy. My arm works normally, and I never had any puffiness that some have had. My fear was not in losing the breast but in how far it had spread. I didn't ask questions because I was so terrified.

"The breast cancer was so well developed that it invaded seven lymph nodes under the arm, and usually if it has reached more than two to four, you are in trouble. I had cobalt treatments from four different directions: my back, chest, top, and under the arm for six weeks for sixteen minutes, five days a week. There were no side effects. I expected bad things, because I had heard them, but I had no reaction. I have had radiation twice since then but no reaction. I have heard of nausea and burning of the skin. I've had x-rays every three months from top to bottom to determine if the malignancy has spread.

"I had the mastectomy in November 1973 and started having back pains in July 1974, which became severe by August. They should have given me a bone scan, but nobody even mentioned that. If they would have caught it sooner, it meant my back wouldn't have eroded so far, but they kept telling me I was all right. I could have had radiation earlier. I have a friend who is a nurse, and she sent me to a bone specialist who couldn't believe that the other doctors had not done this.

"They removed my ovaries, and that did not slow it down. For some people that works, as it stops cancer for about a year. Then my mother found out about Laetrile. My mother had a friend who was given three weeks to live and went on Laetrile and lived another five years. A lot of people are on Laetrile in California. I didn't want to go on chemotherapy, because it is a toxic drug and has all sorts of side effects, so with my parents' help, I went on Laetrile from November through February. The drug is illegal in our country, because they feel there is no proof that it is successful. You can get it in Mexico or here, if you know the right people, but the price has really skyrocketed. They have done studies to show that it can be a preventative, but in my case, cancer had gone so far that I don't know how much Laetrile helped. I am lucky having the tumors only on my clavicle, femur, and liver, as cancer of the lungs is very bad.

"I then got a cancer doctor whom I like very much. He told me I almost died because the toxic level in my body was very, very high. I was in the hospital about a week on chemotherapy and radiation. They use radiation on terminal patients to try to take away the pain. I am now on 5FU chemotherapy, one of the oldest. Some people get a shot every week. My doctor feels I should only have a shot every other week. Some people have their hair fall out, experience fatigue and nausea, but I had none of those. I did lose my hair because of the radiation. I am getting stronger and must stay on 5FU until it is no longer effective. Then I'll use the last drug they have. Unless they come up with something new, I will be pretty much out of luck."

Kitty died a few months later in 1975, at the age of thirty-one.

Tressa (33/33): "No matter what happened, I would still be here."

"They were going to biopsy both breasts. My surgeon said he had decided not to have me sign a consent form. From what I've heard, many doctors automatically have their patients sign this consent for a mastectomy before the biopsy, and the woman goes to surgery not knowing whether or not she'll wake up having lost part of her body. I think the choice should be entirely hers, and her doctor should offer both choices. The additional cost and time are hers; therefore, the choice should be also. I feel I benefited so much from my circumstances.

"So I went in the hospital knowing I was only going to have a biopsy. I wasn't that upset. The moment I knew I had to go for a biopsy, I became very calm; it was wonderful. I picked up a lot of books—I love to read—and got myself into a totally positive attitude that no matter what happened, I would still be here. If I lost my breast, I would still be the same person, the sun would still be shining. I would still be able to love my children, and my fiancé would still be there beside me. My fiancé was taking care of my children and was wonderful. He said, 'No matter what happens, I am here and will take care of you, no matter what.' He is forty.

"I was groggy just out of the recovery room and did not see the surgeon till the next day. He said, 'We did find cancer in your right breast, and I will know more when the lab finishes.' The third morning, he said, 'We did not find any cancer in your left breast, but there is a 50 percent chance that you will be back here within five years to have the other breast removed. Even if we take the right breast, we cannot be sure there will never be any cancer in the left breast. The choice is yours, whatever you want to do. I will say that with women of your size, it would be more difficult for you to be fitted properly if you have one breast removed than if you have two. It would be more difficult in the future to think of having an implant or any type of reconstruction done. It is easier if they are both gone, plus the 50 percent chance of getting cancer in the other breast.' It wasn't even worth 10 percent for me to keep one breast. So I decided to have them removed based upon his recommendation. I have not regretted this.

"The right breast was removed, the breast bone scraped thoroughly, and the lymph nodes were removed. On the left side, the lymph nodes were not removed, just the breast. The first thing I remembered was that I'm here, I'm going to be OK. That was the most important thing to me. There was terrible pain from the surgery, but the minute it didn't hurt anymore, I didn't think about it. I was told nothing about the arms in the hospital. The left arm was fairly OK from the beginning, but I could not use the right arm at all. Both are fine now.

"They found, after examining my report, that I am in the 90 percent cure bracket. There is only a 10 percent chance that there was any cancer remaining, and that would diminish as time went by. So the doctor didn't feel there was any need for radiation as there was no lymph node cancer. I last saw him in October and am to return in six months."

Opal (34/56): "I was just glad to be alive."
"I had a single mastectomy twenty-two years ago when I was thirty-four, and I don't remember if they told me the different types of mastectomies. After surgery, the doctors were at my bedside, a couple of nurses, and the anesthesiologist. I looked at the surgeon's face and he looked so tired, so unlike himself, and there were two bottles about my bed, one with clear fluid and one with blood. I said, 'You had to remove my breast, didn't you?' He said,

'Yes, I did.' Then I went to sleep, but when I started to think about it, I was just glad to be alive. I had given them a lot of trouble during surgery, as they had to stop the surgery for two hours because I went into shock. They told me they almost lost me. I was on the edge and could have gone over. I was thirty-four years old at the time and had two children. I was so glad to be alive.

"You can see my ribs through the skin; there is no flesh there at all. For the first twenty-four hours there isn't much pain, but after that, there is a great deal of pain. Seepage is always there, and the pain would become more extreme. For a couple of weeks, I went to the nurse in the doctor's office, and she kept draining the seepage about every other day. I was tightly banded and swathed in bandages, and my right arm was tied down to my side so I wouldn't pull any sutures, because the skin was rather tightly stitched. Being right-handed, one just naturally moves that hand, so I used my arm some. My upper arm was bandaged to my side, but I could use it to my elbow. The doctor had me keep brushing my hair until I was able to brush up to the top of my head.

"I had a full-time nurse, and my sisters stayed with me around the clock. Doctors didn't know much about the mastectomy then. My vital signs were not too stable because of the severe shock for two days. I was in a semiprivate room with two beds. Follow-up exams consisted of x-rays, feels underneath the arm and around the neck at three-month intervals, and once every six months for the second year.

"I did have radiation for the mastectomy, and it caused my chest wall to be very sore and very weepy. It was well over a year that I was sore. The doctor said I should be glad to have radiation because good cells regenerate themselves, but malignant ones do not, as they are killed by the radiation. During the fourth week, he made this decision, not I. He is the kind of doctor that makes his own medical decisions. He said they thought they got it all, but you can never tell, because one cell may have broken away, and he wanted to take the opportunity to be 100 percent sure. Radiation was for eight weeks, three times a week, every other day, hitting two spots for two or three minutes at a time. They alternated the spots.

"I had to go in for a biopsy on the second breast in 1965—thirteen years later. I was more shook up than I was for the first breast. This time my husband was a fully practicing alcoholic. I don't know why, but I felt real sad for him that he would have to face this. For alcoholics, everything is an excuse. I just felt sorry for him and knew that he would not like to face it. I found this one myself, on the outside of my left breast, the upper outside quadrant. The doctor told me this is called the dangerous quadrant because of the glands that come in from underneath the arm. I felt more concerned this time, but when I got to the hospital, I thought that this would be no problem. It turned out to be a benign cyst. I had more soreness from that biopsy than I did from the mastectomy."

Joleen (38/41): "I have a Pollyanna attitude."

"There was no mammography prior to surgery. The surgeon found a malignant node at the top of my breast. I lucked out in that it hadn't spread to the glands and was caught in the very early stages, so my prognosis is very, very good. I had a modified radical removal of the complete breast, most or all of the lymph nodes under the arm, and the pectoral muscle was left in tact, which is helpful in recuperating. I have been told by technicians and surgeons that I have a beautiful scar, and I think it almost beats having a breast. [She laughs.]

"I knew absolutely nothing about mastectomy. I signed all the hospital papers because of my Pollyanna attitude that I had no intention of having anything seriously wrong with me. I knew I was signing papers for major surgery, but I had not discussed it with absolutely anyone, including my doctor, and was amazed to wake up and find my breast amputated [only woman to use this term]. If I had to do it again, I would do it exactly the same way. I feel this attitude helped me respond positively postsurgery. If I would have known that I could have had a partial mastectomy, I would have grabbed it, but now I don't think that would have been a safe thing to do. I was very, very conscious of my physical appearance and would not have had the full breast amputated. I was only married for six months, and although our marriage has become a very good marriage, at the beginning, it was based on pretty primitive and childish emotions. The physical was a great part of it, and that would have been uppermost in my mind.

"My husband asked what I thought of my surgeon, and I said he reminds me of an astronaut: he flits in and out, is distant and uncommunicative. I don't have the opportunity to ask questions, no empathy, but I'm alive. I've heard he is a good surgeon, but I don't know from my own experience.

"I took the surgery very, very lightly as far as was apparent. A few hours after surgery, I was holding a cosmetic session for the student nurses that were around me. I put up a wall and masked myself, then felt the pain alone. I've always practiced this.

"The doctor told me I should try to raise my arm beyond a ninety-degree angle for three weeks, so I did what I was told. I feel I had a pretty easy time of the mastectomy for several reasons. I have a relatively high threshold of pain, and he managed to deaden the nerves from my elbow to my waist. I felt nothing. I still don't have the full feeling back in my chest wall. I didn't attempt to raise my arm above my head until about two months after the surgery, although I did shampoo my hair when I got home. I raked leaves and did various exercises.

"Another mass was on the other breast two years after the mastectomy. It was fibrocystic disease. We keep a close watch on it and have xeroradiogram every six months, as I have other lumps now. I see the doctor about every three months. They do not discuss the possibility of removal of the second breast with me. I have a pretty good statistical idea, but statistics don't mean a lot to me, in that each case is so variable. I had asked a doctor what the chances were of a cancer metastasizing from the uterus to the breast. Odds are very, very low. The breast to the uterus, yes, but not visa versa."

Alice (39/47): "I was scared."

"I didn't ask any questions. I was scared. Just the word *cancer* scared me. I thought of death. My six children were kind of young—eight to twenty-eight—and the ones eight and ten were at home. My children were shocked, shocked. They thought of death too. My husband has heart palpitations, but he seemed not to be shook up. I am the most concerned about losing my breast, more than the cancer.

"There was no pain whatsoever for the ten days in the hospital. One nurse came and poured out her problems to me, which released me. She had leukemia. I forgot myself. I was depressed, mainly because I did not have a family here. None of my friends came to see me. My two closest friends were having problems with their husbands and were working. Only my husband came.

"I had to endure cobalt radiation—fifteen of them, with the longest lasting for five minutes. I went from three a week, to two a week, to one a week; just on the chest, not on the back. I got burned, but the doctor told me I was light skinned and subject to burn. It had left scars from the cobalt. [I could see the scars above her V-neck blouse.] After the thirteenth one, I got up the next morning and passed out for a couple of seconds, but no nausea. I wasn't tired and went out and did housework every week.

"Follow-up exams were once a year in the doctor's office. After four years, they found it had spread. They put me in the hospital and took out my ovaries, adrenal glands, and did a bronchotomy. I also had cancer of the liver. I live with death and where cancer is going to go next. I'm the type that likes to know what is going to come. Some people don't like to know. I do, because I want to get adjusted to it, really. I don't like surprises. I now drink chemotherapy every Friday and feel fine.

[Alice phoned me several months later to say she and her family were moving back East, and she no longer needs chemotherapy, as there is no trace of cancer anywhere in her body.]

Andrea (39/43): "I feared most losing my breast."

"I have had cancer of the uterus at the age of thirty. It was not removed because of cancer but because of excessive bleeding, and they found it as a fluke, a rare kind. I do not remember the name. Had I not been a doctor's wife, they might not have done as careful a pathology report study as they did. The pathologist told my husband this. They take chunks, slice it up, stain it, and do studies. The cancer was so small, not the kind you would unusually find, and it could easily have been missed on a routine pathology.

"Waiting to go to the surgeon for a biopsy was the bad thing. I feared most losing my breast. I could barely get through the routine of the day prior to surgery. Really not doing even that, just sitting a lot, feeling very sorry for myself, talking it out with my husband, but with nobody else.

"I knew a lot about mastectomy, as I had worked in surgery as a student nurse, had seen it done, had taken care of such patients, but that was as far as the technical thing. They took a mammogram and found some suspicious areas, but the doctor still did not think it was a malignancy. I've often tried to wonder about the surgeon. He was as upset at this point as I was because we were friends. He tried to deny it to himself as well as to me. At the time, I can remember thinking that if he knows something, I wish he would come right out and say so, so that I don't feel like a nut in being the only one that thinks so. He told me years later that he did feel very strongly there was something there, but he could not bring himself to admit it, because we were friends.

"I thought it is too bad that they don't do the biopsy and then have you think about the mastectomy, because that is all I had known twenty years ago. The surgeon did say that there was discussion among surgeons about radical versus simple, but his feeling was that in the area where the lump was, it was safer to do the radical, should it be necessary, so there would be no possibility of leaving a stone unturned. I had a radical mastectomy, all lymph nodes removed, no metastasis. Upon waking from surgery, I remember the surgeon leaning over me, and this really bugged me for a long time because he said, 'Well, Andrea, we had to do the big one.' That just frosted me. I thought, *He can't even say the word.* I can remember feeling a great pressure on my chest, putting my hand up, and then I cried.

"Radiation and chemotherapy were not discussed. I did have linear accelerator radiation afterward. My surgeon said that because of where the lump was, they didn't do what they used to do years ago, because that was super-radical surgery [Halsted: splitting the breastbone and taking lymph nodes out that lay under the breastbone] and is rarely done anymore, particularly if the nodes under the arms are negative, which mine were. But as a safeguard against any malignant nodes that might be in this area, surgeons and radiologists felt that because of the area, radiation would be a wise precaution.

"I went for radiation five days a week for four weeks, three minutes per day on the area underneath the chin, down the center of the body, across the body and back to the center of the chin. Very little side effect except a feeling of a lump in my throat because of inflammation of the tissues. I have known some having cobalt that have had nausea and vomiting. Then I went back once a month until six months were up and then every three months to the radiologist."

Brenda (39/40): "Cancer bothered me; losing my breast didn't phase me."

"He knew I was in the medical profession as a practical nurse. I had papillary adenocarcinoma. *Papillary* simply means 'nipple of the breast,' *Adeno* denotes relation to a gland. 'Adenocarcinoma, malignant neoplasm of cells in glandular pattern, frequently with infiltration of adjacent tissue. Metastasis recurrence after removal is a possibility' [Brenda was reading a report given her by her doctor.] If there was recurrence, I imagine I would be a little shook. I told my doctor that I don't mind losing my breast, because I don't have that much to lose anyway, but I do mind having cancer. Cancer bothers me, losing my breast didn't phase me in the least. Maybe it is because I am small, I don't know."

Julia (39/67): "I didn't like having a breast removed."

"I did not have a lump. After having a baby, I came home and there was so much milk it just flowed all over the place, so they used a breast pump. The doctors attributed cancer to the breast pump. After they dried me up, there was a clear secretion from my breast, and I was concerned about it. My doctor was a pathologist and said, 'We want to watch this very carefully. As long as it is clear, there will be no problems, but if at any time there is a sign of blood, no matter how slight, I want to see you immediately.'

"I was lying on the beach on my tummy and there was the evidence. I'd had a baby in 1931 and found blood in 1946. It was right after World War II, and they couldn't find a bed in the hospital. They finally cleared out the doctor's consultation office and operated there. There wasn't a john, a number on the door, there wasn't anything—just, *boom,* the surgery. The army had not released enough doctors, and the hospitals were just jammed. These were the days before recovery rooms.

"I had never heard of anyone ever having had a mastectomy, never. I didn't know what they were going to do, and they didn't know what they were going to do. They took me in and said there was a possibility that I would lose my breast, but they did not know. I wasn't very happy about that, but I really and truly did not think it was going to be malignant. Very naive, no one had ever done any talking about it, so I wasn't too afraid until I woke up and saw the arm of the sleeve of my husband's jacket and thought, *Uh-oh, he wouldn't be sitting here if everything was all right.* My husband reacted in a very matter-of-fact way. He had been watching [me] for a long time, and I said, 'They had to do it, didn't they?' He said, 'Yes, dear, but you are all right.' So I went back to sleep again. I didn't like having a breast removed."

Donna (41/42): "I cried, got hysterical; it was something important to me."

"You don't eat, you don't sleep, that is all you think about. I cried, got hysterical. My husband was out of town, and I told him to come home. I just about didn't sign the papers when I went to the hospital. That took about two hours longer. I was in such a snit that I wasn't going to sign it. My husband said, 'You sign it; you have no choice.' I said, 'Yes I do have a choice, and I do not want to sign it.' He said, 'I have faith it is not going to be anything, so go ahead and sign it.' So I sat there for about another half hour, much to the nurse's annoyance, my tears running down my face.

"After surgery, I just had to look at my husband to know that my breast was removed. He had a look of sympathy, and that is a look he generally does not have. My sons acted the same way, but they tried to look cheerful. You are so groggy you don't really care at the time. Then I guess I got hysterical, and a nurse came in and gave me another hypo. I kept waking at night, getting hysterical, getting another hypo. I was a very bad girl, I guess I would say, but I was very depressed, wishing I could die and all this. I was very much mad at the world because it was something that was important to me, and I was losing it. I sure wasn't the best patient in the world. I didn't want to eat anything or have anyone wash me. I just didn't want anyone who had to look, and I didn't like the attitude of the nurses, as they had not had it done and could not relate to me. I didn't like someone saying, 'Oh, you are going to get over this.' How do they know? That is their nurse's training to be on duty, but that doesn't mean they are thinking what you are thinking. How can they feel what you feel? I couldn't buy that at all.

"My family doctor knows I'm a sissy, so he has to be gentle with me. I'm like you in that I can't say enough good things about both of my doctors. The cancer was ceracell, the fastest-growing kind. When he told me this on the fourth day in the hospital, I took another nosedive, totally. I had just gotten over my hysterics and said, *OK, Donna, you had better pull yourself up by your bootstraps, and get on with living here.* It never occurred to me that a biopsy report was going to come back. It was living it all over again. I had a good night and thought, *I'm going to be able to cope with this,* and then he came in with the report. It occurred to me that, yes, I do have cancer, and that this may be growing as it is in the lymph nodes, and it is the fastest growing, and it just completely wrecked me for days.

"I did my arm exercises faithfully every day. It hurt, but I was determined I was going to get my arm going. There were a lot of strange pains, spasms, and when I got home, it was horrible to sleep at first. Sitting up was painful, and turning on my side made the pressure hurt more. It took me about five weeks to get my arm above my head. Now, a year later, there are strange little pulling feelings in my chest. The surgeon told me that a lot of ladies had told him it was between six months and a year before these little pullings would go away."

Ethel (41/47): "I didn't want to openly admit it."

"No, we did not discuss the possibility of having a breast removed, just the removal of a tumor. I knew nothing about mastectomies. It was something that happened to somebody else, but I know better now. You read articles that feel women should have a right to decide what is to be done. The doctor should decide what has to be done. I'm glad that my doctor did what he did, although he has apologized a couple of times for taking the muscles, because the cancer had not spread. He said the muscles did not need to be removed in my case, but I'm glad it was done and done the right way, because it leaves nothing to chance.

"After surgery, I remember that I had a chest that felt like it had a hot poker lying on it. The surgeon has followed me for five years, and I am no longer with him. He never gave me a mammography before, because he never thought that much of them until xeroradiography. I'm a different person now. I would have gotten somebody else who didn't keep me waiting so long. Now I have one once a year.

"I was not taped down, but [the doctor] did not want me to move my arm from the shoulder for a week. No problems though. Maybe it is because I am left-handed and I used it more. I didn't know you were supposed to have problems with your arm, until other people told me. I knew about radiation and knew if I did not have to have it, it was a good sign. My doctor showed me my report twice in subsequent visits, that they took the lymph nodes out in groups of three, and there was nothing there. But the first year, I thought he was just telling me this to make me feel better. As each year goes by, I feel better and think maybe he is on the level. I never knew how many lymph nodes I had until Betty Ford had about thirty removed."

Bernice (43/44): "I am a person of faith."

"I thought I knew a lot at the time, but I am finding out that I didn't. I just knew that the breast would go. I did not try to find out more. I probably would not have delved into it any deeper, because I am a person of faith. I figure that it is the job of the surgeon to know what he is doing, so I will go along with him. I did not ask a lot of questions, and he did not go into a lot of detail. I maybe didn't want to know. I had no reason to question what the doctor told me, my head doesn't work like that.

"I remember in the recovery room, they were asking, 'What is your name? Where are you?' and I told them. I reached down and felt my chest, and my breast was gone; it felt all flat. I said, 'Oh, they took it, didn't they?' I remember this nurse saying, 'Yes, dear, they did.' I said OK and went back to sleep. I expected it. I knew it could happen, so it wasn't any big shock to me. I was so interested in sleeping that I don't remember any big reaction.

"I don't recall too much discomfort. I was very numb. I did not feel anything, and my arm was at my side. I had a tendency to hold it as you would a broken arm—across my stomach. All of a sudden, it dawned upon me that I didn't have to keep it there, and it didn't hurt to straighten it out. I did have difficulty raising my arm. Within a couple of months, I started getting the feeling of itching. I didn't even know my back was numb until it began to itch. I asked my surgeon why I was itching, as it was driving me up the wall. He said that itching is the lowest level of pain. It was everything coming back, and that is why I was itching. I had no reason to think that this itching was not normal. He did not think it was abnormal. I don't recall any pain to any great extent.

"When I would exercise the arm, I could feel the muscles but didn't relate it as being painful. It was as if I had suddenly used muscles I had not used—like when you go bike riding and your legs will cramp and hurt because you haven't used those muscles for a long time. That is the same feeling I had in my arm. I could pretty much put my arm above my head before I left the hospital. I could lift it above my head, but not far. I don't recall the surgeon saying not to use the arm or to use the arm. I just went about my normal routine. I can remember the phone was on the left side [of my bed], and I would reach out to answer it, as some of the ladies in my four-bed ward could not get it.

"The ward that I was in was a really great group of gals. One was a seventy-three-year-old lady with a broken hip, whom you couldn't keep down, and she kept everybody in hysterics and broke us all up. Between the both of us welcoming everybody to our room, we became very attached to our room. I think it helped with the two of us having a good sense of humor. I just didn't want to be alone. But then again, when I think of some of the kinds of rooms that you could get into with people who are hard to get along with, that might not be so pleasant.

"I felt the hospital treatment was excellent. I became sympathetic to the nurses because they really have their hands full. I don't think I could be a nurse and put up with some patients. Sick people can be pretty miserable people sometimes. The nurses did a fantastic job. Their attitude toward me was nice.

"The doctor said I could have pain pills whenever I wanted them. I only took one once because I thought if he left them there, I must need them. From talking to other people, I must have a high tolerance to pain, because I always thought I could not abide pain, but through this surgery I'm not aware of that amount of pain. I was on a pump for drainage for two days. It was a nuisance because I had to wheel the machine around when the nurses took me to the bathroom."

Sarah (44/44): "I was hysterical. The breast was important to me."

"I was scared to death. I knew what my friend had been through. She had extensive radiation treatment. I wasn't looking forward to anything like that. I wasn't concerned about having the tumor removed. I wanted it out of there. I probably could have had the tumor removed years ago if I had insisted, but I don't like to go looking for trouble either. Why subject yourself to that if there is no reason. When I found in the hospital that they found cancer and had to remove my breast, I was hysterical. I was yelling and screaming at the surgeon, and he had to close the door. I caused a bit of a scene. I was angry at the whole world.

"My hysterectomy had been no problem at all. I was looking forward to that. It had gotten to the point that I did not want any more children, as I had two teenage daughters, and I was bleeding at least twenty-eight days out of each month. After the hysterectomy, I was absolutely on top of the world, so far on top that no one could touch me. It was different after the mastectomy, and this was difficult for my sons to understand because I was in such good spirits after the hysterectomy, but not after the mastectomy. They had expected me to be the same, and I wasn't. I was extremely depressed for a long time. I am just now getting out of it.

"When I had the hysterectomy, I wanted to be alone. I felt so bad at that time. But this time, I wanted people around. I didn't want to be alone. The horror in the middle of the night is to remember you have lost a breast. When I'm under the influence of anesthetics, I'm in euphoria. There were loads of friends that came to the hospital when I threw a cocktail party on Saturday night. I enjoyed them. It is kind of a lonely place in the world to be without friends and family. I wanted to see my kids. No one questioned their age, and to tell the truth, I told them to lie.

"My arm was taped to my side for five days, and the pain, oh God! I had terrible muscle spasms. The first time it happened, I thought, *Oh God, I'm having a heart attack.* This went on for days and weeks. I did not have to go through radiation or chemotherapy, as there was no lymph node involvement, and my prognosis is great.

"The trauma of living without a breast—the breast was important to me. I might have an implant. I'm not sure if I will have an implant, because I don't know if I can go through another surgery just for cosmetics. The doctor did everything in his power to save my nipple. He said I had a fifty-fifty chance of the nipple living, but it didn't, because it did not have the proper blood supply to live.

"I reacted very strongly to Betty Ford's news release. I thought they went too far when they spoke of her 'cancerous right breast.' It made her sound like a diseased woman, and it hit me wrong. If I had been in her position, I would have tried very hard not to have the details released. They could have said she had a malignancy, and her prognosis is very good. *Disease* sounds dirty, icky. I thought she must have had a pretty sound pain shot to walk out of the hospital and raise her arm the way she did. This is one of the main reasons I called you, because the truth was really not shown there.

"Many people don't realize the arm problems and the pain. I exercised my arm by doing about twenty or thirty jumping jacks—without jumping—and doing about forty to fifty in the evening when I am watching TV. I stopped for three days and could hardly use my arm. Now I do exercise daily. There is a history of cancer in my family. My mother died at the age of fifty-five, and that is pretty young. I am forty-four and don't want to die now. I don't think much about death."

Olivia (45/54): "I don't know why I am crying."

"My surgeon is a man of few words. I remember the discomfort of pain. The nurses were wonderful. My doctor didn't make any suggestions as to what would help mentally. I just burst out crying one day and said to my roommate, 'I don't know why I am crying.' She said, 'For God's sake, ask for some tranquilizers. You have been through hell, and you need some help.' I didn't think to ask for help, and the doctor didn't say anything. When I asked, he said OK, but it was the nurses and a friend of mine (who had her breast removed because her breast kept making benign tumors) who helped me the most. I feel he was a good surgeon, and I am confident that he got all the cancer, but if I could pick and choose, I would pick someone with his ability but with a little more warmth.

"A radical right mastectomy was done in January 1965. Radiation had been discussed and although the cancer was advanced, it had not gone into the lymph glands, so it was up to me. He said he was not recommending it to me but felt it was a safety measure. I had twenty-five cobalt treatments. Did I ever have side effects! I was nauseated. By Monday I would be all right because I didn't have any treatments over the weekend, but by Friday, I couldn't keep anything down. I lost some weight, about fifteen pounds. I hated cobalt radiation because of the nausea, but I felt I was being helped. I was not given very deep radiation, because I had a partial lubectomy with TB years ago. One doctor told me later it was just like having two surgeries. Those twenty-five cobalt treatments gave the same shock to your system as the original surgery.

"A simple left mastectomy was done seven months later in July 1965. This came after I went for my examination. When he noticed there was a thickening in the left breast, he said it might not mean anything, but it is a good indication that cancer might develop. So he suggested that I have it removed, which I did. There was no need for radiation this time."

Beryl (46/50): "I have gone through ups and downs with recurrence."

"I have a history of cysts in both breasts, not a terrible amount, but they are there. During an examination, a lot of cystitis and only one cyst was found. The x-ray showed there was nothing to be concerned about. Then I started to have a tingling sensation in my breast and under my arm, and I became concerned. I was diagnosed as having cancer in my lymph system and was really scared.

"I knew about all the alternatives but didn't have a choice, because it was so extensive. I felt I was in the best hands, and my uncle [statistical research doctor] was looking after my best interests, so I didn't feel I needed to know about the alternatives. I had a radical mastectomy and only have a bony, washboard chest now. I don't know how many lymph nodes were involved, but they told me it was quite extensive. I awoke in a lot of pain, was scared, uncomfortable, and kept complaining. It was terrible, and I reacted the worst way I could. I was able to use my arm right away.

"Fifteen months after the surgery, I have gone through ups and downs with recurrence: two more surgeries, and two more recurrences in these past one-and-a-half years we have been married [second marriage]. Cancer cells had surfaced on my chest as sort of a rash. They removed it in the hospital in just an hour or so as an outpatient. In less than a year after that, I noticed my lymph nodes were swollen in my neck. Every time I go back, there are all kinds of workups, bone scans, x-rays, etc. I'm now on a three-months checkup.

"Then they decided to take out my ovaries, because estrogen feeds breast tumors. If I were lucky, I would have a 30- to 40-percent chance of remission. About one year later, I got sort of a raised area on my chest wall, and they said the tumors were growing again and that the thing to do was to put me on male hormones. So I'm up and down like a yo-yo of stress, wondering when it is going to hit me again. All this time, I am keeping my husband on an even level, telling him that I'm doing fine and everything is just great.

"Then it came back again—two months ago on the same chest wall—and it started to grow again, very small tumors. Instead of doing a surgical adrenalectomy, as they do here in California, they put me on cortisone and thyroid—a chemical adrenalectomy—and I have been on it for two months now. It still hasn't gone away, and I have pain and aches, you know.

"I feel that if I had a better diagnosis by the radiologist in the beginning, this thing would have been caught sooner. I thought I could work with a surgeon in California, but he said he wouldn't unless I did it his way, and he wanted to do a surgical adrenalectomy. They take out your adrenal glands that are over your kidneys, as they also secrete estrogen. Every doctor does things differently, and they don't do that procedure at Mayo Clinic where my uncle works.

"These two women I know, we all had a radical mastectomy, had our ovaries removed, and had our adrenal glands stopped, and their cancer has progressed faster than mine, and they are deteriorating faster. We all have it in our bones but in different degrees. I have it in my pelvic-bone area, as far as the bone scan shows. Chemotherapy is the only drug they have to slow up the adrenal function, it is the only thing that they have. I don't know if I'm going to use it or not yet. My uncle doesn't want me to take chemotherapy, as he feels it is not as successful as it should be. We will cross that bridge when we come to it. They don't give me too much information at any one time; they just put me step-by-step. I'm just scared to death about being on chemotherapy, about having anyone take care of me, being dependent on anyone, of losing my hair, and all the side effects. My uncle tells me [chemotherapy] is all that is left, but that hopefully by the time I need it, there will be something more. No, I've not had radiation."

Grace (46/57): "I can remember how great it is to be alive."

"The doctor didn't tell me about different types of surgery. I was in surgery about seven-and-a-half hours, saw my husband later, and he looked more dreadful than I did, I'm sure. I have been very fortunate in that I have never lived with great depression over cancer. I can remember how great it was to be alive. The weather was late August and lovely—the sun beamed, the birds were singing, and how great it was to be alive.

"This arm swells and has been quite a problem. The first year, the one arm was quite a lot larger. My husband rigged a pulley like they have in the hospital, and I slept on my back with my arm in the pulley for the first year, as my arm had a lot of fluid [lymphedema]. I still do that now. It is still larger than the other. I was determined and got my arm above my head very soon. I would play handball with my little girl. My threshold of pain is high resistance. For in having children, it wasn't bad; I had them quickly and easily, and the contractions were not bad.

"They found nineteen nodes, and one was affected. I do ask questions and am a pest about asking questions. I wanted to be a doctor and went to premed school. It is my body, and I care more than the person examining me. It took a long time to heal. The doctor did not use stitches but crossed the skin some way. The skin was so thin that it kept breaking loose so I didn't wear a bra for a long time.

"I realize there is the possibility of recurrence, but I don't dwell on that or think about it, because I take care of myself. The surgeon told me he had been to a conference, and they felt the newest thing to fight breast cancer was the hysterectomy, to get rid of estrogen, because the question exists that estrogen perhaps causes cancer. If you remove the source of estrogen, perhaps this will cut down on the recurrence of cancer.

"At this point, I am lackadaisical because I have been so well since 1963. If the second one would have to be removed, I would be more panicked this time because it meant that there are cancer cells dormant all this time that might not only take my breast, but my life. The anticipation of what is going to happen is frequently so much worse than the happening itself."

Blanche (47/48): "I just wasn't going to cry and be silly about this."

"I got a terrible headache when the surgeon showed the mammogram and told me everything. Surgery was about three weeks after I discovered my lump. My main worry was that I was embarrassed, because my surgeon did not want to operate without talking to my husband. He wanted his patients to go in with a good understanding and a relaxed feeling, and he wanted to know both husband and wife. I was worried because I don't approve of gambling or drinking, so I never did tell the surgeon that my husband was in Las Vegas. Just told him my husband was out playing golf. I was more worried about being embarrassed to tell him about my husband than I was about my own problem.

"I was sick with a terrible migraine from all these other things. My husband came home about five A.M. from Las Vegas, and I was mad to think that he would go off like that when I really needed someone to talk to. He didn't know and didn't realize that it could be cancer. I was the only one at that time in the hospital for a mastectomy. I preferred being in a room with others so you could talk and not worry about yourself.

"My doctor said he would never operate without a bone scan first, because if he had to do a mastectomy, he wanted to make sure there was no sign of it in the bones. If there were, he would not do a mastectomy but use other treatments.

"I woke from surgery and saw my husband standing over me. He almost broke down, and [he] said they had to take everything and the lymph nodes. I remember turning away at the time, because I didn't want to cry. I just wasn't going to cry and be silly about this. I just didn't want to break down. I have never cried since the operation. That is very strange, because I am very sympathetic and very sentimental over movies, and when children dress up cute, it always brings tears to my eyes. But about myself, I don't cry over anything. I didn't ask all the questions you did. I was so dumb. I just thought, *It has to be done. It has to be done.*

"When somebody gives me a lot of sympathy, I cry. Maybe if I hold back, they won't give me sympathy, so I won't cry. The nurses were great, excellent. I was in the hospital for six days and healed very fast. The only pain I remember was when they removed that tube. I heal so fast that I think some of the skin had started to grow over those tubes. I remember having twitches and would go, 'Huh'—like a deep breath, like pulling a muscle.

"The doctor said he had removed about twenty or twenty-six lymph nodes—not all of them—and I had cancer in one node closest to the tumor. He and my internist decided not to give me radiation, because I have a lot of trouble with asthma, and they didn't want to take a chance of damaging my lungs. They didn't think I needed it, since they got it all, and it was only in one node.

"I was unable to move my arm at first. I got discouraged. I tried to do things they told me, like walk up the wall with my fingers. I would sit in a chair and swing it. Then I would tell the kids to look what I was doing, and they said, 'Oh, Mother, you're cheating and bending your elbow' and would kid me about it. When you got [the arm] to a certain height, it was painful, but no one understands that. I had it above my head in about six weeks.

"I had to go back every two days for two weeks to have the drainage aspirated. They would measure the amount and said this was not an unusual practice. I go every six months to the surgeon, then after two years, I will go once a year. I've had a zeromammogram and a bone scan at the end of the year."

Della (47/52): "Although I am a nurse, I really wasn't expecting a mastectomy."

"The doctor told me the biopsy was benign, but I feel that my doctor was negligent in that the lump had become harder, and he should have sent me for the biopsy about six months sooner because it was suspicious. I really wasn't expecting a mastectomy.

I had asked for a private room but was put into a room with three others. One was having the same surgery as I was, so we talked about it and were both somewhat apprehensive. I then remember waking up, feeling the bandage, and realizing that this was it. It was quite a shock. I can remember that very, very clearly. My thoughts were, *It can't be me. I can't have cancer. I'm too young to die.* I was forty-seven.

"My doctor didn't discuss too much before surgery, because he knew that I understood the process—a frozen section, and if it is malignant, the mastectomy. I was not given any choice as his method was the radical. He didn't give me any alternatives. I would still want the radical, because I feel my chances would be better for survival. I want to see the results twenty years from now of the lumpectomy and the less radicals. I don't believe they have been used long enough to compare the results.

"They removed the pectoral major muscle. I had the most radical removal of the chest muscles that you can have [Halsted]. There is nothing left but ribs, and I can see my heart beating. I was very, very lucky that the muscle that was left in my shoulder permitted me total movement of my arm. So from the beginning I was able to raise my arm straight up, and I have been told by various radiologists that he did a good job on the surgery.

"I know people who have lifelong problems with arm mobility, so I was lucky on that. The nurses helped me move my arm. Everyone expressed great amazement that I could raise my arm up as far as I could from the very beginning. The surgeon always commented that he was pleased with the result.

"I had one lymph node metastasis. That indicated to me that my chances were less good than if I had none, but now that the five years have elapsed, I don't really worry about it anymore. I have had many, many associations over the past years with people who have had the surgery. I know people who have had many nodes involved, who are still alive and doing very well. I know of people who have died, who have not had any nodes involved. I don't feel there is any hard-and-fast rule. I just don't think there is any way you can tell for sure.

"I can't remember the kind of cancer I had. My doctor handed me my chart, in an envelope that was unsealed, to take to the radiologist, and I felt he did this because he knew that I would read it from cover to cover. He did the same thing in the hospital, because he wanted me to have confidence that he was telling me the truth. As for the layperson, no doctor or nurse is ever going to let a patient see the chart. It is an ethical thing that is drummed into you from the day you start. I would never do it. I can't remember the name or grade [of the cancer], only *interductal*. Mine was in the upper, outer aspect of my breast.

"The nurses were excellent and gave me lots and lots of attention. My doctor came twice a day, and I had a lot of support. I was very depressed, so I was glad to get it. I was very concerned that if I died, I would have no one to take care of my three children (ages thirteen to seventeen). I was very, very depressed for a long time—probably eight months.

"I was not able to have cobalt treatment until June because I had so many complications following surgery, and my wound did not heal until October of that year. I had sloughing of black, dead tissue because of inadequate blood supply. Then there was fluid formation in the shoulder that continued for weeks, and I had to go back to get rid of that all the time. I had an open wound about three inches that was a draining, gaping wound for a long, long time. I had to go back to get skin grafts off my abdomen about six weeks after surgery and had two blood transfusions, but the graft did not take. I felt that I should have had blood transfusions before surgery, and the healing might have been faster. I never did ask the doctor why he did not do so, because there was nothing to be done about it now.

"Cobalt radiation was used to prevent the spread of the cells, since I had one node involved. I went twenty-five times, four or five minutes at a time, over two areas—the shoulder and don't remember the other, but not on the back. It made my depression deeper. I was taking care of three children and an ill mother and was still debilitated from the surgery. It was a difficult time."

Margaret (48/49): "As long as there is life, there is hope."

"I had an internist who had been treating me for a growth on my thyroid for about eight years. I asked him to examine my breast because there was a thickness I had found. He said there may be just a little cyst, but he felt it—more to put my mind at ease. When he touched it, he said, 'Oh my God, you have a tumor in there.' I grabbed his hand and said, 'Oh no, you told me it was nothing,' and I started to cry. He said, 'You are a big girl. Now, stop crying,' and sent me to a surgeon. I begged him to do the biopsy right away. I'm that way—when something has to be done, I want it done right now. I'm better in the battle than waiting for the battle. I was examined by three different doctors, and they were all optimistic.

"I told the doctor not to tell me about the lab report: 'Just don't tell me. Don't tell me. Let me go into the surgery thinking— I don't want to know one way or another.' I signed the mastectomy release, but he knew that night that it was malignant. I would rather go into surgery still hoping. If I had known that I was going to lose my breast, I might have panicked that night. Whereas I was still very much uptight, I still had a very high hope since all the doctors thought it was all right. Yes, I would still want it that way.

"I awoke six hours later with tremendous pain—tremendous, tremendous pain—mostly in my back. I wanted to move, but my arms were tied down, and I had an I-V in one arm. The first thing I remember was my husband stroking my cheek. My husband said, 'It is going to be all right,' stroking my cheek, and he was gone. Not real consciousness, just drifting, a mass of pain. Then the woman in the next bed was watching television, and I thought, *I can't stand it; I wish she would turn it off.*

"I asked the doctor if he got it all, because that was very foremost on my mind. He said, 'You would still be down there if I didn't get it all.' But I didn't know anything about lymph node involvement or the dangers, the terrible dangers, of breast cancer. I thought, *If they get it, they got it,* but in many cases, they don't get it all. Cancer is a very deceitful thing. After five years, I've talked to a lot of women who haven't had it for five years, and then it takes off and kills them.

"They took eighteen nodes and seven were involved, and that is quite a lot in the first stages of cancer. I asked him what my chances were, and he said good, that he had just been to a conference where they said lymph node involvement was good because it catches the cancer cells that have gotten away from the primary tumor. He has always been very honest with me, and he said we know so very little and are stumbling around: 'We just have to wait and see, since you cannot predict this disease at all.' I went into deep depression.

"I found a tumor under my arm where I was operated on. The tumor was malignant, four months after my mastectomy. They said, 'We have lost a battle but not the war; we have many things to fight with yet.' You need to emphasize that in your book—that the only way they can detect cancer is under a microscope. They can't tell just by feeling.

"In the meantime, more tumors appeared on the chest wall, about fourteen or fifteen. By now they are not telling me very much because I have been through too much emotionally and physically: three operations, hepatitis, tumors popping out, and I am blind in one eye. It was diagnosed as metastasis in that eye.

"They did not do cobalt because my surgery was too radical, and radiation would burn up the chest, my skin, and complications could arise. They decided to do an oophaectomy—the removal of both ovaries—and they do an awful lot of this in the case of breast cancer. It is to cut off the estrogen. He said that usually when the surgeon removes a tumor from under the arm, they get it all, and 'We will do the oophaectomy because your estrogen flow has to be stopped, as this cancer is fed by estrogen.'

"I asked him what this would do, and he said, 'We are going to take away your femininity, because we are going to take away your estrogen.' He did admit that he could have given me male hormones but felt that the removal of the ovaries was the way to go. It only works in one out of three women. I told him this was a very small chance. I was very upset because this would be my fourth surgery. He said, 'I would do it if I were you.' When I was getting dressed, his nurse said, 'Honey, think about it very carefully, because it is very important, and I think you should consider it.' She wanted me to have it done, so I did in March.

"They told my husband that they did find cancer in both ovaries: very small, about two-centimeter tumors, which they would never have felt by a pelvic-area examination. Also, I had involvement in the skin that covers the intestines. [The doctor] examined my liver manually because he did not trust the pictures, but the liver was fine.

"About two weeks after that surgery, my eyesight started coming back, and the tumors started disappearing from the chest, and within three weeks, the tumors were all gone. The surgeon asked me if I knew how phenomenal the results from the oophaectomy had been, that it was a near miracle. So I thought I had it made. They took away my estrogen, and the tumors are going away, and I am going to be just fine. They did not tell me that this was not a lasting thing. I called the radiologist who told me that this was just a temporary thing.

"They called in a cancer specialist, who told me this was a very serious recurrence, and he could not cure cancer. I asked for chemotherapy, and he said, 'No, because we would never know if the oophaectomy was successful or not, so we have to wait and see.' He said, 'I cannot cure you,' (he said that three or four times) 'but we will try to control it.' He was the one who told me later of the total involvement. If I were average, the oophaectomy would last a year.

"It didn't last a year. On vacation in Europe, I found another lump under the left breast and one under my left arm. I went to a cancer doctor, who sent me for a bone scan, lung x-ray, and liver scan. I asked about a mammogram of the remaining breast, because of the American Cancer Society and everything you read telling you to have one every year if you have cancer. He said not in my case, that if I developed cancer in the remaining breast, they would not remove the breast but treat the whole body. If you have cancer in two or more spots, they have to go under the assumption that you have cancer in other parts of your body, so they treat the whole body rather than one place.

"I went to my urologist who looked and said, 'Now you aren't a girl anymore.' I felt like somebody hit me over the head. Now I have cancer in my bones. I have been on chemotherapy now for two weeks. I am taking the quadruple—a combination of four chemicals. Two are given in the vein once a week, and the other two by mouth daily.

"I am hopeful with this chemotherapy. They cannot cure me; I realize that. I am tolerating the drugs very well and consider myself very lucky. This is a type of control of cancer like insulin is for a diabetic. It does kill cancer cells, but it kills good cells, too, and that is why you have to have blood tests every week. I know of a woman who has been on this drug for five years. As long as there is hope, there is life. The thing that really keeps us going is that someday they are going to come up with a cure or more effective drugs."

Margaret died in May 1975, five months after our interview.

Agnes (48/58): "I did not really understand what was going to be done."

"I had just been examined two weeks before, and it wasn't there. They tell you it doesn't hurt, but it did hurt. There never was any talk of a cyst or anything. [The doctor] told me that I would have the lymph nodes taken out from under my arm, and I didn't understand. He told me that if he found anything, it was all going to go. I was not given any alternatives. I didn't ask questions, because I had a lot of faith in him then, and still do. He knew a lot more about it than I did. I didn't realize what it was really going to be. I thought it was going to be like the radical mastectomy done in April 1964.

"Mammography was used when the second breast started to bother me. I was very heavy, and this one started to hurt. He showed me the report, since I was ready to blow my stack because I thought I was going to have the same thing again. The radiologist said there was no cancer, but there was a tissue change. And in view of my past history, the breast should be removed. The second surgery was done in December 1964, but it was a radical mastectomy. If I had known, perhaps I would have said to take the lump out and watch it for a while. It is such a mess that your personal life just comes to a screaming halt. I did not really understand what was going to be done.

"I never had anything like that before. I was in the recovery room and looked at the clock and saw that seven hours had passed. Then I knew that I wasn't in there for any biopsy. The nurse wouldn't tell me anything. I was getting a divorce. I said to the nurse, 'Well, I had it, didn't I?' She wouldn't say anything, but I heard her say to the other nurse, 'She knows.' I didn't really react to it—didn't understand it for a long time. If I had to do it over again, I would not have this done. I would take a chance on it because it hasn't been much of a life now anyway. My psychiatrist said, 'Don't you realize that because it is up high, it goes right into the lymph glands?' I hadn't thought of that before. Maybe the surgeon was right and I was wrong. He said mine was a single cell, infinitesimal. I don't know if he told me the kind of cancer I had.

"The only one that encouraged me or even told me about exercises was the surgeon. He made me stand against the wall and walk my fingers. No one told me, either one way or the other, not to use my arm. I don't remember how long it took me before I got the arm over my head.

"Do you know anybody that has gone as long I have and keeps getting spasms? I still get them after ten years. When I go to back out of the car and turn my head, the whole thing goes. And when I get uptight talking to someone, I have learned to control it so it doesn't show on my face. My doctors said it is just nerves."

Becky (51/51): "Mine was a good experience."

"I am a nurse by profession and fully understood my surgery. The night before, my surgeon and I discussed our philosophy and what would happen to me. We agreed that if the radiography were as definitive and indicative as it seems, and the front section confirmed this, I would at least suffer from some form of radical mastectomy. I would lose the mammary and the lymph nodes in the auxiliary. If there were no nodes involved, there would be no need for the super radical. If there were nodes involved, they would have to do the Halsted radical, and certainly, I would agree. I would leave that to the judgment of my surgeon. I chose him and trusted him. There is no way that I could make that decision. I chose a man who is qualified to make that decision for me.

"What we are discussing here is that of modified radical, which usually should be sufficient to its cause, followed then by radioactive materials and chemotherapy. This would depend upon how many nodes he found affected. Two nodes, such as in the case of Betty Ford, then I would assume that he would do only the modified radical and follow me with radioactive materials and chemotherapy—one or the other but not both, or both. After the frozen section, you have the benefit of many opinions—not just the surgeon's—as to the course of treatment.

"I have no recollection of much after the surgery. I experienced very little pain intellectually, compared to what I thought

I would. I was very pleased and not at all in pain in the true sense of the word. I felt very uncomfortable—bruised and battered, like I had been in a fight or knocked down by a truck—but I found that dealing with my pain or discomfort on a twenty-four-hour basis, the pain decreased. The second day, I washed my hair. I was not told not to move my arm. I remember moving my hand with my other hand, because I was not able to move it much. Gee, I wish I had brought my door to you from Palm Springs, because I had a marvelous chronicle of that event, of raising my arm above my head and marking the door to show my progress. Mine was a good experience."

Judy (51/53): "When God is ready to take me, he is ready to take me."

"I had an exam in March and [the doctor] didn't find anything, but in April I found a magazine that showed you how to examine your breast, so I examined myself and found a small lump about the size of a pea. We went on vacation, and I forgot all about it. In September I examined myself and found it was the size of a walnut. It didn't bother me in particular until [the doctor] told me, 'I may have to remove your breast.' I didn't show any concern until I got into the car, and then I bawled all the way home. It then became just another operation, as I'd had a gall bladder surgery, a heart attack, a leg in a cast, and everything was just piling up. Another operation just scared me half to death, even though there is no cancer in my family history.

"The internist suggested a mammogram. Then we went to the surgeon, who explained that the best procedure to save my life was to have the breast removed. There was no question in either of our minds but that was what we were going to do. I knew it might be a modified radical because the doctor told me, but I didn't expect to live, because of my heart. I resigned to the fact of the mastectomy. When God is ready to take me, he will take me.

"When I awoke I felt beautiful, I was alive and found everything beautiful. The only thing was that I couldn't reach. My doctor walked in and then walked out because I found everything beautiful. He didn't expect me to be sitting up laughing with my two daughters and my sister-in-law. My doctor encouraged me to use my arm. He said that before I left the hospital, I was to have my hand above my head. I did after five days.

"My surgeon said, 'I have gotten it all, and you will never have to worry about it again.' I asked my doctor that I understand it can get in your bloodstream and pop up anyplace else, and he said, 'Yes, it can.' Now, one doctor tells me it won't, and another doctor tells me it will or could. He said, 'You smoke, and it will probably be in your lungs first.' Radiation and chemotherapy were never discussed. I do not know what kind of cancer I had.

"My nurse had a mastectomy, and you couldn't tell. She was very large-bosomed, and you have that feeling when she bent over to make the bed, and she didn't even feel like she has a mastectomy. She was very sympathetic, patted me on the back, said, 'Don't worry about it, now; I've had a mastectomy,' and I felt that if she can look that good, so can I. I wasn't depressed about having it removed. I was alive, and that's all that mattered to me. I had some depressions, off and on, but most of the time, I was feeling up.

"There were follow-up examinations to the surgeon for the first six months, then to my doctor who tested my liver and gave me a Pap smear. The doctor felt around the area where the scar was and did a general exam. Nobody told me to examine the other breast, but I do."

Beatrice (54/55): "The second surgery was a real shock."

"I had mammograms and went to my gynecologist, who assured me that it was nothing but a cyst. For a while my internist watched me every six months. Now my gynecologist has my yearly checkup. But I noticed the cyst was getting bigger, located on the breast at 'two o'clock.' I had a noncancer-related hysterectomy twelve years ago, but [the surgeon] left the ovaries. A couple of years later, he put me on premerine for hot flashes and irritability. It seemed that the cyst would bother me more during certain times of the month, and I noticed during the several years when I decreased my dosage of estinyl, the lump would go down a little bit.

"In 1973, during my gynecologist examination, I told the doctor that the lump was larger and hurt all the time. He said that when I felt it had grown to let him know and he would put me in contact with a surgeon who would aspirate it, because a lot of times there was cancer underneath and you can't feel it because of the cyst. I went home and cut down on the estinyl and the lump got smaller. I asked the doctor if I could have a smaller dosage of estinyl, and he said, 'Well, take it every other day.' It was all right for about a month, and then it started to hurt again. I had a cyst on the other breast, also. My left side hurt but not the right side.

"My gynecologist was out of town, so his nurse gave me some names. I called the internist's nurse and asked her advice. Some names she would not comment on and some she said were excellent. I made an appointment with a surgeon, and he didn't seem too concerned. He, too, thought they were cysts. He said I could go three ways: (1) wait and see; (2) take a mammogram and wait, then take another mammogram and have it aspirated; or (3) you could go in and have it biopsied. That was the surest way, so I said, 'Let's go for the biopsy.'

"I had to go see my mother first in the rest home, and I didn't want her to know about it, as she is ninety-five years of age. So I went in the following week. I just thought it was going to be a biopsy, since I had checked it all these years. I was just so sure. My sister had a real radical surgery [Halsted] in 1966. She also had her ovaries taken out afterward and also had skin grafting that did not take. She had radiation, but I wish now that she did not even have the operation, because it had spread beyond the operation. My sister died in 1968—a year and a half after surgery.

"I signed the paper for whatever would be necessary. I had faith in him that he would do what he thought would be right, so he had permission to perform whatever operation would be necessary. I went in because my left breast was bothering me, but when I came out of it, my right breast was gone. I realized that the bandage was on the right side instead on the left, and I thought, *What in the world went wrong here?*

"He said they made the biopsy on the right side first and sent it to pathology and had been working on the biopsy on the left when the report came back that it was malignant. And he was so sure that this was benign, but they found cancer under the small cyst. He did the modified radical and removed the lymph glands and left some muscles. It was a shock, but I thought they caught it in time. They said the left breast was benign, so they sewed me back up again. I had a Hemovac—a tube that extends down from the side below the incision, and they tape the tube to you, which is attached to a round vacuum to draw drainage.

"The second surgery was a shock. The night before I left the hospital, the doctor came in to see me, and said, 'I'm sorry. I have bad news for you.' Four pathologists kept reviewing my frozen sections of the biopsy, and they came to the conclusion that there was a definite pattern there, and the left breast had to come off also. He was going on vacation so he scheduled me two weeks from the time I left the hospital.

"That came as a real shock. I had gone in thinking I would come out smelling like a rose, then . . . I guess I was still in a state of shock from the first operation, and I don't think it really hit me. But when he said the left one had to come off, I was really stunned. So when I went back for the second operation, I was really scared. I didn't want to go back. I just figured my number was up.

"*Cancer* is a scary word, but I went back. Only three weeks between operations, so I wasn't really in tip-top shape to have another surgery. Both were modified radicals, and my surgeon does not prescribe radiation unless it is a question of saving a person's life, or unless it has spread to the lymph glands or other parts of the body.

"They simply found cancer. He told me, but I can't remember the kind of cancer I had. He did say it was not the kind that spreads fast like my sister's. No lymph node involvement for me, and thus no radiation. I was in the hospital seven days for the first surgery, six days for the second.

"I didn't think the hospital staff paid enough attention to my exercises. It seems to have been left up to me. The doctor said I was to start climbing the wall with my hands, ten times every hour, on the hour, for ten hours. The nurses wouldn't even come and tell me to do the exercises. I started it when the Reach to Recovery woman came and showed me the kit. She was very nice, and I was amazed at her recovery.

"I was discouraged at my progress when I got home, because I had slipped back and was unable to reach what I had been able to reach. My arm was not taped down. There was mostly indifference. During the second operation, a foreign nurse seemed to be more interested. It was two months before I got my arm above my head. I didn't drive for about two weeks."

Nan (55/59): "Losing the breast did not bother me that much."

"There was no lump. I was finding a difference in the breast contour. There was no discussion of a mastectomy or radiation or chemotherapy. I kept telling them it was cancer. I opened my eyes after surgery to see a nurse standing over me. She said, 'You don't want me to lie to you.' I wasn't surprised. Losing the breast did not bother me that much. They removed all the lymph nodes. What surgery did not kill, radiation killed. I had cobalt for three-and-a-half weeks, every day, nine minutes a day. They never told me if cancer was in the lymph nodes, and I didn't know enough to ask questions. I may have kidney infections, and my arm is twice as big from fluid buildup, as there are no lymph nodes for drainage.

"One nurse had a mastectomy and told me she still couldn't turn on her left side—hurts even now. I had no therapy whatsoever. The arm is painful, but I pick up the phone with my left arm. I'm bitter about that; something could have been done. I've had twelve surgeries in my life, not all related to cancer. Since 1973, I've had cancer in the pelvic area and had surgery for removal of the gallbladder and a cyst big as an egg in the liver.

"I didn't want cobalt anymore. I had side effects—burned me through and through. I had a lot of allergies and my skin is sensitive. Now I'm on chemotherapy—four different chemicals. I have carcinoma in the tissue, the worst one to control, as it will travel faster than any other. There is 30 percent chance of survival. Side effects could be blood clots, pneumonia. My doctor was very honest. He knows I've been through a lot, and there is no reason to cover up. I had a liver and bowel biopsy and go back in six months for a bone scan. I would never have the radical again.

"I am weak with big red splotches all over. The splotches do not itch. I'm not to lift anything, not even a pot of stew. I'm not to bend the spine more than [necessary], for when cancer goes to the spine, the spine could break. I'm also on a mild tranquilizer and can't do any work. I take chemotherapy—two kinds intravenously once a week on Monday, two kinds orally every other day, huge shots of vitamins once a week on Monday, plus a blood test every Monday. I sleep a great deal because I'm anemic."

[Nan was so ill she phoned and asked if I could interview her on the phone, which I did. A few months later, I again phoned Nan to see how she was and was told by a new tenant that Nan's husband had sold the house and had moved to Texas after the death of his wife. She could not say exactly when Nan had died.]

Glenda (55/55): "I didn't cry. I just accepted it."

"Waking from surgery was a little unfortunate because I would have liked a little time to adjust to waking, but my daughter is on the staff and was in recovery with me, and I awoke in tremendous pain. The nurse explained they had to awaken me completely before they could give me another pain shot, as there is less risk before other medication is given. My daughter was standing there, and she meant well, but she did not realize that I was not equipped at the moment to hear. If it had been later in the room . . . , but I was in pain and the nurse was preparing a shot and my daughter said, 'It is all over.' I said, 'That is good.' She said, 'You are all right; we are in the recovery room, and it is all gone.' I said, 'What do you mean?' She said, 'They took it all off, and you know they had to do that.' I just wasn't equipped at the moment and it hardly registered. I was also connected to the Hemovac after surgery.

"I didn't cry. I just accepted it. It was just at that moment of awakening, wanting a little time to be in a better state of mind. I just had a real acceptance of the whole thing. I didn't fight it at all. If this is the way it has to be, then thank God, it is all over with. There was some lymph node involvement: don't know exactly how much, but several out of twenty-three. There were two small lumps. I have not been psychologically ready to look at the pathology report. The doctors seem quite competent, and my daughter saw the report.

"I think I picked up a bug after I started chemotherapy tablets. After two days, I became extremely nauseated, had gastritis, and spent a miserable night. He said there might be one person that would have this type of reaction, but it was the smallest possibility. They had never had one instance of this before, and he questioned me closely to see if there could have been any other cause for it. I feel all right now. I take tablets five days; then I've had a bone scan, blood tests, chest x-rays after surgery."

Denise (56/57): "Is it over, or isn't it?"

"I had carcinoma cancer. It had not spread at all, and I did not need radiation or chemotherapy. However, I do have a blood clot on my arm—on the top above the elbow—and it is quite a good size. It hurts and is obvious, as it is swollen. I discovered it shortly after returning home from the hospital. It is a lighter area of skin. I keep my arm elevated, and at times it hurts. It is just part of after surgery. I just accept it. [Denise started to cry but said she didn't want to cry.]

"I still cannot open cupboard doors as I do not have the strength. I can raise the arm elbow-high, not shoulder-high, because it starts hurting. This puts my hand about two inches above my head. Part of the inability to use the arm is because of my back surgery. I have a lot of muscle spasms. I now feel a tingling from the nerves of the mastectomy, especially in cold air.

"Awaking from surgery I thought, *Is it over, or isn't it?* Then I started feeling and felt the bandages. My family doctor had prepared me, but the surgeon hadn't. I do not recall too much in the hospital. I was given codeine, but I became allergic. I wanted to talk to somebody about the mastectomy, but the nurses didn't want to talk to me about it. They were nice, but there was no discussion about it. I am too reserved to ask. I wish I was more open, but I'm not. I'm trying to break away from that. I knew what had happened to me, but I didn't know exactly what to expect as to the outcome. I wasn't aware that I couldn't do anything for weeks with that arm."

Vanessa (56/60): "I did not collapse or fall apart."

"I had no knowledge about the mastectomy. This is what made me bitter. I didn't expect my breast to be removed. You are so numb. I had tubes, and when you went to the bathroom they went with you. Five women had the same surgery that night, and the nurses asked if I would go see them, because I did not collapse or fall apart. It was the year of donors of lungs, kidneys, etc. I kidded that I had a breast to donate but that no one wanted the damn thing because it was too small. I said, 'I'm lucky. What about those who have big whoppers?' They all laughed.

"There were no lymph nodes involved. The doctor said the only regret he had was that he had to remove a vital nerve. I'm still numb. About two-and-a-half years after surgery, I had such pain that terrified me. It was just nerves trying to get back. If I had known that—if it were someplace in a book—it wouldn't scare you half to death. Even to this day, I get small stabbing pains, but now I know what it is.

"The surgeon had said that if I wanted radiation, I could, but he said I really didn't need it. I didn't heal well, and it started to smell. The other women I had started to visit had their bandages changed. They had different surgeons. My MD said, 'If the surgeon doesn't change it soon, I will.' There is a difference between an MD and a surgeon. [When the bandages were changed,] I did not want to look. I didn't want any part of that, but the fresh bandages did make me feel better.

"Nothing was done about my arm in the hospital, but the doctor told me constantly to reach when I go home. I had the project of reaching for the light above a painting in our house to turn it on every night.

"Now I have x-rays once every six months. It had to be done. I was terribly grateful. Nobody had cancer in my family. I just accepted it; there was nothing else to do. Women who don't go to see about cancer are just stupid. I had a friend who almost bled to death because she was afraid of cancer, and it turned out not to be cancer."

Clara (59/71): "I reacted terribly; the attitude was that it just can't happen to me."

"I was having an examination for a cold, and the doctor found a lump. About two years before, the reumatologist found a thickening, about pea-sized—very, very small—and told me to watch it. There was no liquid found upon aspiration, and no mammography was used. I'm a registered nurse, and it never struck me that it was malignant. It was Christmas week. I had an appointment the following Wednesday to have my hair done, and I didn't cancel it. I just went in to have a biopsy.

"I reacted terribly. I'm trained in how to take care of people. Some nurse told me in the recovery room, and I just reacted terribly. I couldn't believe it because I wasn't prepared. With all my own background, it should have entered my head that it was possible when the doctor didn't get any fluid from it, either that or I just blocked it off. In looking back, the attitude was that it just can't happen to me. I have talked to nurses, and we all seem to have this attitude—that it had happened to all of these people, but it can't happen to me.

The way it was done [breaking the news of breast removal]: He stood at the foot of my bed, and I said, 'You did a radical,' and he said, 'Yes, it was cancer, but we got all of it, and you don't have to worry.' Then he turned and walked away. I spent the ten or twelve days in the hospital in a state of suspended numbness, and he never talked to me about it. He never said anything. A lot of people came to see me and were very good to me and brought flowers. I had a surgeon who was just a cold-blooded fish. I got a staph infection, but they let me go home over Christmas. I am the only person I know in my personal life who had the bad medical treatment I had."

Daisy (59/62): "If you have to do it, then go ahead and do it."

"I always had my doctor examine my breasts because of the fact that there had always been cancer in my family. The mammogram showed cancer. I was shocked but didn't cry or get all unglued about it. I felt that if it was there, something had to be done, it had to be taken care of, I was in the best hands, and they were going to get all of the cancer. I was secure in that feeling.

"I had known about the mastectomy, as this was only four years ago [1970], and there was more talk about it. The idea of having a breast removed did not appeal to me, but if it meant having my health . . . . and the thought of the children came to mind. If I could just have some more time to live, I was very happy about it. I really didn't have any fears. I wasn't afraid. I worked with a woman who had a mastectomy. My surgery was about four days after the discovery of the lump.

"I didn't feel that I was going to die, since I was in good hands. I had great confidence in the doctors. They were very reassuring doctors, explained the operation to me very thoroughly. There was a lump in the right breast, and they didn't know if it has spread to the left breast. There was no lump on the left breast, but in the original mammogram, the technicians felt there was a slight shadow, and they would also do a biopsy on the left breast at the same time. Just before I went into surgery, he said, 'I may have to remove your left breast, also.' I said, 'If you have to do it, then go ahead and do it.'

"I knew they had removed both breasts, there was no doubt in my mind. Let's put it this way, the Man Upstairs had prepared me. I had a very spiritual experience that night before my surgery. In a bed next to me, there was a woman who was very active in her church, and her minister came as she was going in for surgery. I was lying very quietly in my bed, the curtain was drawn, waiting for the intern to come in for me to sign the papers. The minister was reassuring her and didn't even know he was doing just as much good for me as he was for this woman. It calmed me down. I just can't tell you the feeling I had; it just calmed my fears. It just gave me peace, so when I woke up and the doctor said, 'I'm sorry. We had to remove the left breast, also,' I said, 'That's all right. I knew it.'

"I couldn't move my arms. This upset me when they brought my tray of food. A young Black girl brought me a tray in the evening and said that I hadn't eaten very much. I said, 'Nobody helped me; I can't pick up anything. Would you mind feeding me?' I was able to get a few spoonfuls in my mouth, but it was an effort. I will never forget. I was determined to try, but she was marvelous, so great. In fact, she helped me through my exercises and everything that came after that. She was encouraging me to lift my arms to my chin, then the mouth, then eyebrows. And I really worked at it as she kept after me. She was a great inspiration.

"I had radiation treatments in the area surrounding the breastplate to make sure as a precaution. I had eighteen treatments and maxitron under the right arm. Maxitron is the next step up from cobalt, like a laser. I had no bad reactions to it whatsoever. The reaction was my own doing. I had a fear of the machine. I made the bad mistake of looking up at this huge machine. Here you are with your arm back of your head, they mark a target, and I did just fine for the first two treatments. The third treatment, I got very nervous, thought I moved, and had a terrible fear of the machine. The doctor reassured me that she watched every move, so I didn't worry about it. I had fifteen max-itron treatments to assure the lymph nodes were free. The maxitron was for less than a minute and the plain x-ray about three to four minutes. This went on for six weeks to two months, three to four days a week.

"The only reaction under my arm was to destroy the hair fol-licles. There might be a fibrosis condition that may develop under this arm, but the doctor said you won't know, and I have no feel-ing. A fibrosis is a hardening of tissue as the three- to five-million volts that go through your body will make a scar tissue. The only problem on my chest is that capillaries came to the surface of the skin. I got quite a burn from that, and it is still sensitive, but it gets less sensitive as time goes on. But it took three years before it got to the point where it really didn't bother me."

Robin (60/62): "Having faced the issue, I was ready to go on."

"It was the day before April Fools' Day, and I hoped it would fool me, but it fooled the doctor instead. I awoke and found my breast gone. I knew, inside, it would be so. I had faced [the fact] before I even went in. I was frightened of cancer because I had lost my mother and grandmother to cancer. I was frightened, but when I came into the hospital, I was not too flabbergasted about it. Having faced the issue, I was ready to go on. In fact, I was on my feet and down the hall soon after surgery. Meantime, I was doing these exercises, yes ma'am! They didn't have to come tell me about them, because I wanted the use of my arm.

"My husband was at sea at the time. He is a merchant marine on an oil tanker. I knew he was coming in and tried to reach him by cablegram that I was going into the hospital. He knew I had the lump, as he had called me from one of his ports, and I had told him that the doctor didn't think it was important. He got off the ship while I was in surgery and was disturbed about my physical condition, but not disturbed about the fact that I was having a breast removed. It didn't bother him.

"I felt very good, no pain—not physical or mental. I felt very good. I visited others in the hospital, comparing surgery, etc. Most of the women were frightened to death about it, but I wasn't. I think they were frightened by the knowledge they did not have. Before the surgery, the doctor had discussed radiation and chemotherapy, but none was necessary then. I am now on chemotherapy because the cancer came back on the scar tissue one year later, and in the neck. I have been on pill chemotherapy for almost a year, and it is almost gone. I keep checking for symptoms, then go to the doctor. He did remove the cancer on the scar tissue in his office. They are taking excellent care of me."

Bertha (64/64): "I felt I had taken care of myself."

"I have had a physical examination once a year for many years, so I never neglected things. On May 28, my doctor didn't find anything. I don't know why he didn't find anything, but in less than three months, there was a noticeable change. One breast began to be distorted, more of a flattening or hardness, that is all that I can describe. I was having shots of fire going through—a dull sort of pain, but none of it bad enough to complain, exactly. The doctor said that if it was hurting, it was benign because cancer doesn't hurt.

"He took me on Monday, had the mammography, operated on Friday, and it was quite a mess. Cancer was in all the lymph glands. I wasn't disturbed about losing my breast but about how far the cancer had advanced. I felt I had taken care of myself. I also don't know the kind of cancer I had.

"After the modified-radical surgery, I was most comforted to find my husband standing there right beside me. It seemed that I had no sooner closed my eyes, than my husband said lunch was there. He said there was a hamburger, and I said, 'For goodness sake, you eat it.' But I did eat all the custard he fed me."

Heather (64–65/66): "Resignation. I'm more or less resigned."

"I went to the doctor, who asked if I had always had the in-turned nipple. He suggested a mammogram. I was very apprehensive, as I had several friends who'd had breast cancer and were dead. I didn't know much about breast cancer except for the experiences of my friends. The mammogram showed there was a lump and the possibility of cancer. No doctor explained mastectomy alternatives.

"It was rather grim, in that I went in one time to have a biopsy, went home, and then had to come back to go through the whole thing again. To feel that it was benign, then having a high like that, then to be told you had to go back, was shattering. I knew when I awoke that the breast would be gone, since I had been in twice. I remember a terrible feeling of listlessness, which is not really the word. *Resignation* describes it better. I'm more-or-less resigned. [There is] a feeling that there are things I want to do before death—accomplishment.

"I have asked what kind of cancer I had, but I am not positive about what the answer was. There had been reference by the doctors of radiation and chemotherapy, but in terms of 'let's see how things progress.' I do not know if the cancer was in the lymph nodes. I had physical therapy to regain the use of my arm, and it was several months before my hand was above my head.

"Later I had a pimple or something of that kind on the left breast. The doctor said it was nothing, but it might be a good idea to take the other breast. I went to my internist and he agreed with the surgeon. It really was more or less a practical matter. My husband and I thought it would probably be wise to have the second breast removed. Just a simple mastectomy. The pathology report showed that it was negative."

Martha (78/79): "I very seldom cry over anything."

"The drainage was quite heavy. They changed my bandage five or six times a day. When they first changed it, I saw the scar. It looked terrible—one of the worst things I have ever seen. I never cried during the whole thing. I very seldom cry over anything. I hold things in. I thought he butchered me. I didn't say anything to him about it.

"I had to have radiation for ten weeks, four minutes, five days a week, of cobalt. I had a ball in the hospital and in radiation because I got along swell with everybody. That sounds crazy, but I did. In the hospital, I took all the pain pills then walked all over the hospital. I had a lot of company; all the nurses were nice. I'm one of those kind of people, I guess, who gets along with what I have to. There was no reaction to the radiation. The doctor said I had a 10-percent chance of it coming back, and he wanted to make sure.

"I don't know what a lymph node is or if he took them. He didn't explain, and I didn't ask, because I didn't know what to ask about. I brushed my hair practically right away. There was no pain, but I fell and broke open my wound. My daughter and good neighbors helped me."

Marie (42/42): I was well prepared for any outcome.

I had signed a consent form prior to surgery because my surgeon had thoroughly discussed various mastectomy options. I sought additional information from libraries, a friend showed me her mastectomy, and books were loaned me by our family doctor from his personal medical library. I contacted two other surgeons for a second and third opinion. The surgeon I chose said he does not perform the extreme Halsted, because current scientific evidence shows that the modified radical mastectomy was as effective and less deforming, thus offering a better quality of life to the woman.

The one-step biopsy was my choice. I was admitted to the hospital, given a general anesthesia, and a biopsy tissue sample was frozen and examined in the pathology laboratory under a microscope. The surgeon and his operating staff waited to hear if cancer cells were evident. A modified radical mastectomy was immediately performed, as the lab report indicated cancer in the left breast.

I was well prepared for any surgical outcome and was not surprised when I felt my chest and found my left breast had been removed. As a Christian, I knew I would awaken in one of two places: here on earth, or in my Father's house. Either would be His will for my life, and I trusted Him.

Anesthesia always takes me into deep, deep sleep from which I waken very slowly. I was aware of the loving presence of my husband, but his words were not penetrating my mind. Just seeing his dear face after surgery, I knew that God had blessed us again. I fell back to sleep with a feeling of absolute joy. I was alive to be with my beloved husband!

Pain was well regulated by medication, and my left side was numb from surgery. My left arm was taped down to my side, and I was attached to a Hemovac machine by a small tube inserted into my left side through a tiny incision. There was no pain caused by the Hemovac, but I had not been told about this possibility. I was disturbed by the noise from this machine as it drained fluid from my body. The combination of the noisy Hemovac, the tube entering my body, and my arm being taped to my side, made me feel helpless in being dependent upon a machine. My thoughts centered around the concern of what would happen if this darn, inanimate object malfunctioned. A nurse assured me that the Hemovac was quite safe. Even so, I never did make friends with that Hemovac, but I'm not comfortable around any medical machine that hovers over me.

I had asked for a private room because I wanted time for quiet reflection after surgery. My colleagues at work understood and honored my request that they not visit me in the hospital. They instead showered me with flowers and encouraging cards, which were greatly appreciated and brightened my spirits. It was a time when I wanted only intimate friends and family around me.

The hospital had a magnificent view of the ocean, but beds are placed facing toward doorways instead of toward windows. My surgeon explained this was done because the hospital administration had conducted a study and found that patients seemed more comforted when they could see human beings pass by their rooms, particularly at night. This became so understandable one night after my family had left.

For some unremembered reason, I felt anxious, rang for the nurse, and asked the young girl if she would please just hold my hand. I assured her I was not in pain, just needed the touch of a human being, and proceeded to apologize for taking her away from other duties. There remains such a vivid memory of this young girl, who was not a nurse but a nurse's aide. She held my hands, speaking softly as she encouraged me. Our conversation turned to her needs, and we, in turn, were comforting each other. A lovely memory.

Equally memorable is when a friend came unannounced, took my hands in hers, and proceeded to manicure my nails. This was her precious gift to me. Sometimes we all forget the importance of touch, and after a mastectomy, touching is particularly valued because the woman is being told she is loved for who she is, not for what her body was.

My forty-third birthday occurred five days after surgery. I was comforted when my family brought a birthday cake to my room, because that assured me they were fine. I had the habit of sending my mother flowers on my birthday, thanking her for being there when I was born. Now she was in my hospital room when I was again given life by God.

A few days after surgery, my surgeon came to tell me and my husband that lab reports showed cancer in five lymph nodes of the many that had been removed for biopsy. This information was difficult for both of us to hear. I felt depressed, discouraged, and weighted down by yet another hurdle to cross. My husband calmly assured me that we would face this together, and I smiled, knowing this would be true.

My surgeon explained there was scientific controversy concerning which was the best treatment when cancer enters the lymph nodes: radiation, chemotherapy, or a combination of both. In my case, he recommended radiation as a safeguard in case any remnant of cancer remained. I agreed but told him that I would stop such treatment if radiation proved more harmful than beneficial to my recovery.

I never had the habit of freely moving around a hospital after previous noncancerous surgeries, but stayed quietly in my room recuperating, following doctor's orders. I thought I was again to remain quietly in my room after the mastectomy because of being attached to the Hemovac and also because of the fact that my arm was taped to my side. No one told me differently. I did drag that Hemovac to the bathroom with the help of a nurse or her aide.

One day a nurse angrily barked, "Why aren't you moving that arm?" I replied that I would ask my surgeon when I could begin exercising, as I knew immobility would make it much more difficult for me to use my arm later. That nurse's scolding was graded one step below the Hemovac in my esteem. My surgeon later explained that my arm was taped to my side because he did not want me to use it for a while. I don't remember when the tape was finally removed or when I was given permission to start exercising my arm. I do remember the surgical tape caused an allergic skin reaction, which was uncomfortable for a time.

A few days before being discharged from the hospital, my surgeon said he would be in the next morning to remove the bandages. I spent a restless night thinking about that event and found myself more anxious than I was about the surgery itself. Despite all the research I had done prior to surgery, I envisioned a huge circle being left on my chest where the breast had been "sliced" off like a piece of bread from a loaf. Fear brought dark, illogical thoughts to mind. I fervently repeated two words over and over again, until I finally fell asleep: *trust God.*

The morning arrived, and in walked my surgeon with his usual cheery disposition, saying that it was time to remove the bandages. As he reached with his right hand, I blocked it with mine, saying, "I'm not ready for this; I'm not ready to look." He again reached with his right hand, and I again blocked it with mine. He allowed me for the third time to block his right hand, then sheepishly removed the bandages with his left hand.

We both broke into laughter at his trickery, and for the first time, I gazed upon my scarred chest where a breast had been. There was a very neat wound, which would heal with time. Relieved I said, "Oh, I can live with this." He said, "I have left my initial on your chest—look, an *s.*" I laughingly agreed and reminded my surgeon that with the help of God, he had saved my life and that the *s* on my chest would forever remind me of this.

My surgeon then said that I might want to consider an implant. I stammered, "Do you mean they can make a breast to match the one that is left?" He laughed and said, "Oh, Marie, only God makes them that big." As we continued our laughter, I thought, *What a splendid human being he is, and how wonderful to be able to genuinely laugh after so many weeks of stressful anxiety.*

He explained that I would have to have reduction surgery on my remaining breast in order for an implant to match. I was repelled by the idea of attacking a healthy breast after just having one removed due to the disease of cancer. An implant under these conditions was unacceptable to me. Although I grieve the loss of my breast, my life is more important to me than having it.

Cobalt radiation began several weeks after I had returned home and was administered over several weeks, with minor side effects. My skin became more sensitive, like having a light sunburn after lying at the beach. I applied dry-skin lotion, and this problem was solved. Resulting fatigue was the most bothersome. I was able to drive myself to the treatments and work half-days as a school administrator, but my energy level was depleted after each cobalt session.

The fear of the radiation machine and of being placed in a small room (slight case of claustrophobia) proved more problematic to me than the treatments themselves. I concentrated on turning my thoughts to positive images and laughed as I reminded myself that I may never make friends with any medical machine.

Long-term side effects of radiation were not discovered until years later when I needed a chest x-ray for flu symptoms and was told my lungs are scarred from the cobalt used. It has been suggested that perhaps my enlarged thyroid and recent heart murmurs, due to two faulty heart valves, could also have been caused by the radiation treatment in 1974.

My surgeon, my husband, and I did what we thought was best at the time, given the information available. There is no second-guessing on my part today, and I have no regrets. How can we argue with having my life extended these past twenty-five years? My life will end one day, in God's perfect timing.

We Are Women Who Prepared to Face Our Futures

Entering our hospital rooms with foreboding, we left deeply grateful for our lives. We realized that the mourning process over our loss was just beginning. What would we encounter as we returned home to resume our lives—lives forever changed by the removal of our breasts? What further challenges would we be asked to meet, endure, and overcome? We had already encountered cancer and challenged it by our willingness to undergo surgery and treatment, which called for every ounce of strength within us. As women of courage, we continued to embrace life, and many of us followed our faith through trust in God.

"They that wait upon the Lord shall renew their strength; they shall mount up with wings of eagles; they shall run, and not be weary; and they shall walk, and not faint."
—*Isaiah 40:31*

"And now, Lord, what wait I for? my hope is in thee."
—*Psalm 39:7*

"For thou art my hope, O Lord God: thou art my trust from my youth."
—*Psalm71:5*

"Be of good courage, and he shall strengthen your heart, all ye that hope in the Lord."
—*Psalm 31:24*

"We can never be certain of our courage till we have faced danger."

—Duc Francois de La Rochefoucauld
French author and moralist (1613–1689)

5

BADGE OF COURAGE

"Jesus wept."
　　　　　　—John 11:35

WHEN WE FIRST VIEW OUR SURGERY, emotions are as raw as our incisions, and tears are often shed. Great effort must be exerted, both mentally and spiritually, to remind ourselves that we can ultimately adapt to our scarred body. However, not all women are able to accept their changed appearance.

Coping is a complex process. Women who seek quality of life will see a positive side to tragedy. Women in danger of "poor psychosocial outcomes, tend to use three strategies for coping: crying and becoming desperate; taking tranquilizers and alcohol; and [saying] other people are far worse off."[1]

Adjustment to surgical disfigurement exposes varying attitudes. Some women seek flight through adultery, threatened suicide, divorce, or denial, which allows fear and shame to paralyze them into inaction. Other women choose hope through acceptance, marriage, faith, and reaffirmation of life through a positive self-image.

We seventy women coped with our loss using behavior similar to that described above. Our reactions ranged from an obsession with our scar to an observation that it is only a scar. Most of us chose hope through our faith and self-acceptance, thereby affirming love of life despite our loss.

Bernice (43/44): "I wasn't aware of what I looked like to other people."

"I remember looking down and seeing the scar in the hospital when the doctor came in to change my dressings. I thought it was pretty ugly. I began to wonder how that doctor knew how much skin to leave so that it would meet. I do sewing myself, and it would be just my luck to cut too much off on one side and not have it meet, and I kept relating to that.

"I was a little sad but don't remember crying. I cried when I got home about a month after surgery. I went through about two weeks when I just couldn't seem to pull myself up. When I was really crying all the time, I asked the doctor, and he said it was OK to cry, "For after all, you have lost a portion of your body, and you can mourn that if you like." I don't remember crying in the hospital, because I had visitors, and I was trying to keep thank-you notes up for the flowers. There were so many things going on, that by the time I settled down, I was so exhausted, I would fall off to sleep. I didn't have time to ponder or have much alone time.

"The day I got home from the hospital, I went upstairs to change into a pretty nightgown and looked into a mirror. That was the first time I saw what I really looked like still bandaged. That was a real surprise; the mirror in the bathroom at the hospital did not allow me to see below my collarbone because I was so short. So I wasn't aware of what I looked like to other people. When I got home and saw a breast on one side and flat on the other, I thought, *Oh, you look so weird, and all those people saw you like that.* My stomach took a flip. You look so terrible; why didn't I cover myself up when all those people came in? Then I thought, *That is the way it is going to be, lady. Adjust to it.* But it was a surprise because I just wasn't thinking about what I was looking like to other people."

Alice (39/47): "I felt like a freak. I'm more used to it now."

"It doesn't really strike you until you see the scar there. The hardest adjustment is at home. I got into the state of not wanting to see anyone. I felt like a freak. That was my reaction. I had a friend that had a mastectomy a year ago, who is very outgoing and knows a lot of women with mastectomies. I knew no one. I thought it was something you should keep under cover, something to be ashamed about, really. I feel lonely. I can't talk to my husband. It is not his nature. He has heart palpitations." [Alice started to cry.]

Sarah (44/44): "I'm more used to it now."

"I asked to see the scar in the hospital, but the surgeon said there is nothing to see and changed the bandage so fast I didn't see it. I saw it on Tuesday. It was ugly. I looked in the mirror and it was awful. I felt deformed, really. I got bathed, got dressed, and went to the market. I'm more used to it now. My sister has seen it, but she is a nurse and was looking at it in a different aspect than I was. The lovely lady selling the prosthesis saw it. No man has, as I am not going with anyone now."

Donna (41/42): "I just don't like the scar. I think about it every day."

"Two times a day you shower, and so you think about it when you dress and when you undress. I have never looked at my scar fully yet [one year after surgery]. You can do amazing things with a towel. I don't want to just stand and glare at it. I don't have to look at it. If I can dress and put on my prosthesis and look like a normal woman, fine, then I don't have to look at it. Oh, no, my husband has never looked at it, and he never will. I don't think I am going to be able to look at it. I don't really see any reason why I should. I feel I'm pretty normal, but I just don't want to be reminded of it twice a day.

"You had said you would come over to my house to interview me, but my husband would be home, and I just didn't want to talk in front of him. I don't want to talk about not looking at myself in front of him. He thinks I should have looked a long time ago, and occasionally he will say, 'I think you should.' He thought it was pretty much of a hang-up with me. I guess it was, but I don't get hysterical about it or anything. My doctor feels I'm blowing it all out of proportion."

Jennifer (27/27): "Oh, it is a shock when you first look at it."

"I looked at my scar in the hospital by removing the tape in the corner of the bandage to look. I don't know, I had to look. Oh, it is a shock when you first look at it. When the doctor came in the first time to change the bandage, I just shut my eyes and said, 'I'm not ready to look at this yet.' It doesn't hit you that you had a mastectomy until you look at yourself in a mirror. I don't know if that was your reaction, but when you look in the mirror, and there is no boob there—I think I cried. That was the first time I really got depressed, and it really hit me."

Opal (34/56): "It will improve."

"I first saw the scar when they first changed the bandage in the hospital. There were sutures, and I didn't think too much about it. It doesn't look too hot at this stage of the game, but it will improve. I was swollen and couldn't tell what my chest would be. My chest is just barely covered with skin, no flesh whatever [Halsted radical]. I really wasn't shocked. I don't recall how I reacted."

Glenda (55/55): "It can't be my body."

"I saw the scar at home. I just couldn't believe it was me. I felt sort of displaced, as though this was happening to someone else. It can't be my body. My first thought was, *I can adjust to this.* A younger woman probably would have a more difficult time adjusting to this, but I am fifty-five. I accepted it stoically."

Tressa (33/33): "How can anyone else look at me?"

"To get over the horror of what I would look like with a double mastectomy, I looked in the mirror at the hospital the first chance I got. The bandage was there, and I thought, *I can't bear to look at myself. How can anyone else look at me?* After the doctor removed the bandages, I went home, and the first thing I did was look in the mirror. Oh, I just went to pieces. To me, it was looking at a monster, not my own self. The stitches were still in. Is it really going to be like this? I had never experienced anything like this double mastectomy."

Robin (60/62): "My scar is there, but it is my badge of courage."

"I faced it right away and looked at the scar in the mirror. My husband said, 'Let me see it.' I said, 'Oh, it is terrible.' He said, 'Let me see; it is only a scar.' I told him to look at all this hangover; and he said, 'You are fat anyway, and it always hung over your bra.' Well, he is right; it doesn't go away. My husband and I have never been concerned about the scar."

Vanessa (56/60): "It was my first surgery."

"I knew that I couldn't take that—looking. For about a week, I kept my back to the mirror after I got home. It was my first surgery, and I didn't want to see the scar. I looked about three or four days after I got home, and I deliberately watched. I had cold chills. It was pretty bad to look at a wound like that. It shakes you up. My husband is a very gentle, kind person. He saw it when he changed the bandages, because I was so tired for so long, so long."

Ethel (41/47): "It was something you had to look at eventually."

"I didn't look at the scar at the hospital. I didn't want to see what it looked like. I wasn't ready for that. I had a mental image of what my chest would look like—a lot of scars burned, like a big hole or slice. He left the bandage on one week longer than necessary, because I told him I was not ready to look at it yet. It was something you had to look at eventually. What I thought it would look like [compared to] what it actually looked like was a pleasant surprise. It wasn't one of those things you take a quick look. I don't remember how I felt. There was no discussion of implants. I wouldn't want to go through that, anyway. The more you can stay out of a hospital, the better. If it is a case of life or death, OK. But cosmetic, no."

Blanche (47/48): "I have to live with this the rest of my life."

"I saw the scar probably the second time I went to see the doctor. He asked me if I had seen my scar; I said, no. He asked why not; I said I didn't know. So he made me look. I said, 'Oh, it is a scar.' (I guess most surgeons are proud of their work.) That is when it kind of hits you how lopsided you are. I thought, *How funny looking. I really look funny now.* Then I really got concerned about it—how I would react. I just kind of swallowed and thought, *Well, I have to live with this the rest of my life.* The only thing is when you get up in the morning, you can't run around the house in your robe without the prosthesis."

Andrea (39/43): "It was not very pretty, but it wasn't as bad as I thought."

"I first saw my scar in the hospital when he removed the stitches, the day before I went home. He told me early in the morning that he would remove the stitches later and that if I felt up to it, he would like me to look. I would have to face it sooner or later. He was very caring and gave me a couple of hours to think about it. He said it was usually a very traumatic experience and that maybe here in the hospital, I would have time to get over bad feelings and tears, quietly and peacefully, if I wanted to do it alone.

"When he came back, I really didn't know up until that moment if I was going to look or not. I decided, better now than never. I looked, and it was not very pretty, but it wasn't as bad as I thought. I cried. Something overcame my tears, because he started to remove the stitches, and I could feel nothing—a pressure, but not a normal skin sensation. I was anticipating discomfort. He said that when they go in under the arm, there are a lot of nerves there, and inevitably some are going to be destroyed. No matter how careful one is in sectioning the tissues, there is bound to be nerve damage. He is right, and to this day, I have no feeling. I can stick myself with a pin and not feel it."

Olivia (45/54): "I had cried before, but not when I looked at the scar."

"They wouldn't let me see the scar at the hospital. When they changed the bandages, I would look down, and they would say, 'Oh, you don't want to look at this mess.' I saw it at home and, oh, it was not a pretty sight. I had cried before but not when I looked at the scar. I don't know why I cried before. I never cried again. When I lost the second breast, I didn't cry."

Brenda (39/40): "My girlfriend had a fantastic sense of humor."

"Being a nurse, I knew what the scar was going to look like. When the doctor came in to change the dressing, I asked if I could look, and he said yes. I looked and said, 'Oh, dear God.' All the stitches are in, and it doesn't look all that great. My girlfriend had a fantastic sense of humor. She came in that night and said, 'Let me see. Let me see.' We went into the bathroom and I showed her. Her sense of humor helped me through. If you are alone and constantly think about it, you could depress yourself. I didn't."

Beryl (46/50): "For about a month, I would dress without looking."

"I just said I was so ugly. I couldn't look at myself and would dress without looking. I was so depressed. Now in retrospect [four years later], it wasn't all that horrible, but then it was horrible. For about a month, I would dress without looking. I just couldn't look at it. That's funny; I had forgotten all about that until you mentioned it. I haven't thought about that for years, but it was a long time before I could stand to look at myself."

Judy (51/53): "I think I'm going to break that mirror someday."

"I thought it was ugly then and I still do. People who have seen it said it was the most beautiful job they had ever seen—told this by my sister-in-law, nurses, and the doctor. I think every woman should take every mirror out of her bathroom. Every time I get out of the bathtub, I just squirm. We have this great big, huge mirror; you can't get out without looking, and I think I'm going to break that mirror someday."

Jeannette (43/52): "The scar was just another scar."

"I have had many other surgeries. The scar was just another scar. It was very neat."

Marie (42/42): I could live with this; I am alive.

Lying down and seeing the mastectomy in the hospital is far less shocking than standing in front of your mirror at home. This full view brought an intense sadness, even though I was no stranger to surgery and scars. How could I not weep for my body and its loss?

I knew that wounds heal with time. My greatest concern was how my husband would accept this scar, as he personally never had any serious illnesses, let alone surgery. There was no reason to be fretful, as he remained his compassionate, loving self throughout this ordeal.

My mother had flown out to be with me. Since I was not able to raise my arm very high, she helped bathe and dressed me. Mom was saddened by the scar, but not repulsed. I drew courage from her caring. Where I was impatient and frustrated, Mom showed patience and calm. I remember thinking, *This is how we must feel as babies in our mother's wombs: warm, safe, protected, and loved.*

Scars are not beauty marks, but because of my scar, I will live and continue to be loved by God, my family, my friends, and yes, myself.

> *"Weeping may endure for a night, but joy cometh in the morning."*
> —*Psalm 30:5*

> *"Blessed are ye that weep now; for ye shall laugh."*
> —*Luke 6:21*

"Children, look in those eyes, listen to that dear voice, notice the feeling of even a single touch that is bestowed upon you by that gentle hand! Make much of it while yet you have the most precious of all good gifts, a loving mother. Read the unfathomable love of those eyes; the kind anxiety of that tone and look, however slight your pain. In after life you may have friends, fond, dear friends, but never will you have again the inexpressible love and gentleness lavished upon you, which none but a mother bestows."

—Thomas Babington Macaulay, First Baron
English author and statesman (1800–1859)

6

ENCOURAGING
OUR CHILDREN

"God could not be everywhere, and therefore
He made mothers."

—Jewish Proverb

THE CRISIS OF CANCER IS MULTIDIMENSIONAL. Each family member begins to cope as best he or she can to the stress, depression, and anxiety that accompanies this disease. Young daughters and sons do not fully understand what is happening to their world. Adult children reflect the same range of emotions that their mothers do: denial, fear, and acceptance.

Mother returns home from the hospital with her life and appearance forever changed by the mastectomy surgery. Her weakened body and fragile self-image require family love, care, understanding, and encouragement. Most of all, she wants to be accepted and reaffirmed by her family as being the "same old mom."

Experiences as Mothers Returning Home

Reactions of children, ages three to thirty-five, ranged from unawareness to shock to concern to fear. Mothers attempted to deal with their own emotions as a woman and wife, while doing their best to walk their children through fear and apprehension.

Kitty (29/31): two daughters, ages three and nine.

"My oldest daughter did not have a particular reaction, because she knew that Nana, my mother, had the surgery and Nana is walking around and fine, so she had no particular fear. I told her that I had a cancerous tumor, and they had to remove my breast like Nana to make me better, and she said OK. Both my daughters have seen me nude, and I can't remember any particular reaction. It didn't bother me at all to undress in front of them, and there was no trying to touch or question."

Alice (39/47): three sons and three daughters, ages twelve to twenty-eight.

"My six children were shocked, shocked. They thought of death too."

Denise (56/57): three daughters, ages twenty-one, thirty, and thirty-two.

"One son died three years ago of a heart attack, and two years ago, our second son passed away from a blood clot on the brain. We have three living daughters. Two have accepted my surgery very well, but not my thirty-year-old daughter. She unwrapped my bandages in the hospital and looked at me, but none of the others have seen me. They are all girls, but they can't stand to see the scar at all. My youngest was nineteen then, and she said, 'Mama, I can't stand to see it.' My oldest daughter is a nun. She did come to visit, but with reluctance. When they did not wish to see, I did not pursue the subject. They loved me and were concerned.

"I'm not ashamed about it at all. If people want to ask me questions, I speak very freely about it. But I do not volunteer anything, nor do I make a statement. I hear a lot of ladies sit and talk. I just sit and do not make a comment. They do not know I have a mastectomy. With my son passing away just two years ago, perhaps with time I will be able to speak more clearly with the two oldest girls. I can now talk very freely with the younger one, but she still doesn't want to see it."

Glenda (55/55): daughter and son, ages thirty-two and twenty-nine.

"My daughter is a cardiopulmonary therapist who helped me find a surgeon, and she saw the mastectomy report. Unfortunately, my son seemed to have the most difficult adjustment of all. He was shattered. He thought Mother was indestructible, for one thing. He has not completely accepted that this terrible thing could have happened to Mother. He is the one that has needed the most help. As he sees me going about my business—driving the car, cleaning the house in a short time—he feels maybe it is not so bad after all. I learned later that he just completely went to pieces, and he is not a weak person. I think it was the fear of cancer."

Tressa (33/33): daughter, son, stepdaughter, and stepson, ages twelve to fifteen.

"My youngest daughter was not interested, but the fifteen year old wanted to forget about it because it was not pleasant. They knew I had been sick but did not understand the emotional thing I had been through. The fifteen year old was the most upset. I sat her down to explain to her, but she didn't understand. She was curious at that age: 'Did they really take them off? How did they do it?'

"When the scar healed, I showed her. She watched me do my exercises. I don't believe in keeping things from children if they are curious and want to know, unless it would upset them to a greater degree than it would be beneficial. She was very shocked, upset. I thought it wouldn't register in a child, but it did.

"My children do not know that kind of pain, hurt, and they can't relate to it. I would definitely show her my surgery again if she wanted to see. She said, 'You be careful and not let the boys see you.' And I said, 'I will.' She was just beautiful but was concerned about getting it herself, as she is fifteen. I told her the probability of her getting cancer was very slim and she wasn't to worry about it.

"I had both girls watch the *Why Me?* film on TV, and I started them on breast self-examination to be aware. I felt they left something out of the *Why Me?* film—me, a woman who loses both of her breasts. To me, it was something different. If you are going to show a little of this and a little of that, how about showing a little about me? You personally relate to that program and look for your circumstances, such as who is closer to me, etc."

Ethel (41/47): daughter and son, ages fourteen and twenty-three. [I interviewed both children.]

Son: "She was only in the hospital for a week, and she didn't look worse for the wear. We had this rig in the bathroom for her to exercise. I knew it was hurting a lot, but other than that, it was just a trip to the hospital. I was seventeen at that time. I never spoke of it to my friends, since nobody every brought it up, and I saw no reason to."

Daughter: "I was eight years old and don't remember anything. I see her now and am used to it, but I hope it doesn't happen to me."

Margaret (48/59): daughter and son, ages fourteen and thirteen.

"My daughter came in to help me change the bandages and would look at it and say, 'Mom, I think it is getting better.' So she was very encouraging. Without my family, I could never have done it."

Grace (46/57): four daughters, ages nineteen to thirty-two.

"I can remember my two oldest daughters standing at the foot of my bed with tears running down their cheeks. They were not sobbing, as they are very controlled young ladies."

Blanche (47/48): daughter and three sons, ages fifteen to twenty-two.

"I have not shown the boys because I am bashful, shy. A couple of times, my daughter has been in my room, and I tried to show her. She didn't want to see, just giggles, and runs out. My children react like I do, just like nothing had happened. My daughter [fifteen] is quite immature for her age, and it didn't bother her. When they come by and tease me by pinching my arm, I joke that they just pinched my handicapped arm, as there is no feeling there, and they just laugh about it. They are very open about it."

Della (47/52): daughter and two sons, ages thirteen to seventeen.

"My children were not too aware of what was going on. We had lots and lots of company and people bringing in food, so the children rather enjoyed the excitement."

Esther (44/57): daughter, age thirty-five (son died at age twenty-six).

"My daughter was concerned and glad that I was well. One of the best therapies was my granddaughter."

Brenda (39/40): daughter and son, ages eighteen and twenty.

"My son was eighteen at the time and wanted to see my scar, so I dropped my robe a little and he said, 'Oh,' and that was it. My daughter was sixteen and did not want to see at that time, but now she has. I've never discussed it with her, but it gives her the shivers a little bit. I've told her to examine herself, but nothing else. I just feel she steers clear of the topic."

Beryl (46/50): two sons, ages twenty-four and twenty-six.

"I wasn't married at the time and had a son living with me. He was upset, worried, and frightened too. I remember that he wrote me a really neat letter, telling how much he loved me and how sorry he was that I had to go through this."

Judy (51/53): two daughters and two sons, ages twenty-six to thirty-five.

"My daughter teased me that one hung low, and that made me feel better, knowing that we could joke about it. I was so happy just to be alive."

Mabel (41-47/53): daughter and son, ages twenty-six and twenty-one.

"My son was nine and didn't realize, until the second surgery, what was happening to me. My daughter is not the kind that talks to me about things, but she does have six-month examinations at the Strang Clinic in New York, where they just do breast examinations."

Elaine (52/56): son and two daughters, ages fifteen to twenty-one.

"The children were very brave but scared because they might be orphans. My son's school grades slipped a bit. They depended on their mother quite a bit. The doctor said they were the bravest children ever."

Lucy (35): reactions to her mother's modified mastectomy in 1966.

"My mother was a registered nurse, an operating nurse. Her father's father had cancer, and her sister had a brain tumor and a mastectomy. Mom was very shaken—apprehension rather than fear, concerned about cancer more than cosmetics. She had taken care of her sister for six months, and this frightened her. Dad was upset. Mom is the strength in the family, and Dad always depends on her. This was her first surgery, and she had a good frame of mind.

"I was glad it was over, but was apprehensive to look at the incision. I can't stand to have blood drawn. Mom is strong. Dad is glad to have her home, as he is easily frightened by things he doesn't understand. I asked Mom how she felt as a woman. The scar was ugly, but she sees herself as a woman, and was not horrified as expected. Mom has a zest for life, is cool, controlled.

"I find breast self-examination very difficult—afraid to find something, feel it is almost inevitable to find something, which is stupid. Hoping it will all go away. I understand intellectually, but emotionally I can't handle it. I'm less fearful now. It is a toss-up between fear of losing a breast and fear of cancer. I could accept cancer of the cervix easier than cancer of the breast. My husband fears obesity in me more than loss of a breast."

Bernice (43/44): adopted daughter, age nineteen.

"My daughter, Dora, was aware that I had lumps before, so it was not a traumatic thing, and everything happened so quickly that neither one of us had time to think about it or become too uptight. My main concern was that she was going to be left alone in this house. That is kind of scary for her to have a mother in the hospital, not knowing what was happening. She seemed to be handling everything all right. She didn't seem to be overly concerned, worried. Maybe that was a front. This would be interesting to find out."

[Bernice asked me to interview her adopted daughter, Dora.]

Dora (19).

"When Mom was to have the biopsy, she came across to me that there was nothing to worry about. When I waited in the hospital and it was taking so long, I figured that is what they had to do. She was so pale, and I was really worried and concerned. It was kind of scary. I went back the next day and we both cried. I told her I was really sorry and worried about her.

"It didn't make any difference to me because she is still my mother, no matter what happens to her. The idea of it didn't bother me except I hoped she would be all right. I hoped that would be the end of it.

"The first time she showed me her scar was when she was in the hospital. It was really puffy, but you can barely see the scar now. No, I guess it was not in the hospital but at home. It wasn't really shocking to me; it didn't bother me.

"Yes, I have thought about having breast cancer myself. I've told people I would rather die first and have said all kinds of things like that. But when it came right down to it, if my mother could go through it, I probably could too—with the help of people who love me. You think of a woman and you think of her anatomy, which is wrong because it is what is inside as a person that makes the woman. But that is hard to get sunk into your head. I don't mean suicide. I just meant that I would just rather not go in and check and find out.

"I'm scared of doctors. I guess I fear the idea of what they may have to tell me. I went in last year, the doctor told me I have a lump, and to come back to see him if it changed. He felt it was probably a cyst, since I am only nineteen. I don't even want to go to find out. It scares me, just the reaction of other people. You look at yourself now, and it would be an awful change. It wasn't an awful change when I saw my mother, but it would be if it were me. I guess it if doesn't change her, it wouldn't change me. I don't examine myself every month, just sometimes. I don't think about it every month.

"A large bust on a woman is kind of an outstanding feature. It would be a greater loss to her personality than someone with a smaller bust. Same if you had long legs. You notice a woman more if she has a larger bust, you pinpoint her bust. If she has long, beautiful legs, you drop to the legs. It would change the kind of clothes you can wear. In the younger girls, their clothes are more the braless type, but in an older woman it wouldn't.

"Mom tried to keep herself active at home by knitting. But I noticed something beginning to happen to her, that she was beginning to get very, very dependent on me after it wasn't necessary anymore—to do little things for her that she could be doing herself. I thought, *Uh-oh, she is going to grasp and not let go.* But then she snapped out of it. What worried me was that she could do some of these things for herself, but was she going to keep clinging? It was selfish of me, but it would be better for her, too. It would put me in the spot of having to live here longer, and I am at the age of moving out.

"She is the same old mom two years after the surgery, but she talks about the mastectomy too much—more than I think she should. She makes me feel she is dwelling too much on it, but maybe it is because it is something she has had done to her, and it interests her. Maybe it is because I have a fear of it and don't want to hear about it. It is great that she is working through Reach to Recovery, because it strengthens her in herself to help others going through it.

"Your book should talk about prosthesis, radiation, and other after effects. Also, clothing and bathing suits. I'm very interested in implants—how they look, feel, and how it is done.

"I asked mom about sex because it seems to me that it would be uncomfortable, and she said, no. The pressure of a man laying on you, would it be an uneven type of feeling? Would you leave the prosthesis on, etc.? If someone likes you for you, it is not going to make any difference to them. A person judges themselves harsher than another person judges them. I find that with myself.

"Oh, yes, I would definitely tell someone I was dating that I had a mastectomy. If someone didn't know, and they happened to reach down there [she laughed], it might be a shock. It would be easier to tell them. I would tell if our relationship got kind of serious. I would feel very bad if a man would stop calling me after he found out I had a mastectomy. But then again, that would be saying that it was more your body he was interested in than you as a person, so it would be better that way. The rejection would hurt, but I would be hurt if anybody rejected me for any reason. Any kind of rejection is pretty rotten.

"Maybe my will to live would overcome my will to die. I don't think that anybody wants to die. There is that will to survive. I am attending a church of spiritualism, and they look at death as going into another world. This is interesting. Maybe there is something very great to look forward to and death is not the end. I like that idea. You can grow in your soul outside your body, because your body hinders you because everybody has hang-ups about the body, but if you get rid of the body, you still have your soul.

"I wouldn't want to be in the bad position of Mrs. Betty Ford and Mrs. Happy Rockefeller, because to have the whole world involved in your personal life is not right. It should be with people who care and are involved with you. I would prefer that the whole world not know.

"I'm letting you interview me, because I thought it would make Mother happy. I've done a lot of things against my mom: the things that kids go through, the rebellion part of it. I'm beginning to come down from that, and I've decided that there are other people I have to consider besides myself."

Becky (51/51): two daughters, ages eight and thirty.

"My little eight-year-old daughter was allowed into my hospital room by the head nurse, who was wonderful. She came to my bed and said, 'How much did they take, Mommy?' I told her the whole breast. She said, 'Don't worry, Mommy, it will grow back.' 'No, honey, it won't.' She started to cry and said, 'I want two breasts, I want two.'

"My whole family has a terrible affection for my breasts, you see. Both of my children have put their fingers down between my breasts, patting me. I have always had the kind of chest that children like to cuddle with, warm and inviting, the rocking-chair kind of thing. My friend was there and explained to my daughter that she could either have me with both breasts but maybe lose me, or have me well with one breast. When you get down to it, you have very little choice if you want to live.

"Then one day, my little girl walked in again and said, 'I want to look at that thing.' I showed her once more, and she said, 'That is ugly; it is gross, and it is a shame that you have to lose it.' With that, she turned and walked out. I felt that was good that she could accept it and could depend upon me not to react adversely. To be perfectly free to criticize what she thought, was good for her. I was glad that whatever groundwork I had been able to lay was adequate to her need."

[Becky asked if I would be interested in interviewing her thirty-year-old daughter, Tina, while she remained to listen.]

Tina (30): daughter of Becky.

"My first concern really was for my father and my eight-year-old sister. I felt that, emotionally, my mother was a very strong woman. She needed our support, most definitely, but she was needed by a small child at home and a husband who wasn't enough educated and responsive to the surgery to realize that this was what was necessary. He acted in disbelief: why her, she had spent her life in helping people with cancer and this can't happen; it is unfair, as she has given her time to other people, and it was unjust.

"As far as surgery, if that is what saved her life, then this is what was important to me. We wanted mother, not a breast, which was totally irrelevant. Her scar was beautiful, and I still think it is quite lovely. He did a beautiful job. We felt very lucky that the muscle was retained. My mother and I are both V-neck people. I don't like turtlenecks. My mother had a very full shoulder and breasts and looks pretty in an open neckline. She looks like the rest of us in her clothing.

"I have had ovarian problems since I was sixteen and have always gone every six months for a Pap smear, and now I will go every year for mammography. I have already scheduled the first one. I use breast self-examination and have since encouraged my friends to do the same, asking if they know how to do this. I realized how very few girls do breast self-examination, because they don't realize and they think this is no big thing. If it happens to me, I hope I can be as strong as my mother.

"This experience was not easy for any of us, because my biggest concern was my sister and father. The word *cancer* to us is very frightening, because cancer and death are so closely related in people's minds. I have a sister that needs a mother for a good many more years. I would be prepared to take care of those needs for her, but it is not the same. If it happens to me, I would want to live to see the fulfillment of my children growing, and be a grandmother. I would immediately elect to have the surgery.

"I have a pretty sexual, sensuous husband who is like all American males and who thinks the breasts are the neatest. But I also have stretch marks from being a nursing mother, and they are not what they used to be. [They laugh and her mother says, 'He still sticks around.'] He still likes them that way, and it would be an adjustment for both of us. We have watched the film *Why Me?* twice together, cried together, and discussed it at great length, and realize this is a possibility for our lives. But it will do nothing but bring us closer, as did our mother's surgery.

"My husband and father-in-law have seen her scar. This is fantastic because my mother is a fantastic person who said, 'I want you to see this,' and she opened her robe. I'm sure this is a shocking thing for a man to see, but these two are now prepared. If this should ever happen to me or my mother-in-law or to my daughter, we now have two men in this world a little bit more prepared, and not letting it become something grotesque to them.

"We have discussed, at one time, all the girls walking down the street with their bosoms bobbing and braless, which I am quite free to do if I choose to, and talked about the reaction men would have if mother walked down the street with one breast bobbing. That might be quite interesting [she laughs]. I don't know how you would approach the man on the street, except through his wife, possibly by educating thousands of them and doing films.

"I saw the show *Why Me?* late at night. Then the next week, I saw another film, which I myself was totally shocked in seeing, about girls in prison and showing a lesbian rape that was the most sensuous thing I have ever seen. I sent my eight-year-old daughter out of the room because I could not believe I was seeing this. I wrote a four-page letter to CBS, telling them how I felt—that emotionally and culturally this was unacceptable. I could go the rest of my life personally and never learn about a lesbian rape, yet something that is important and lifesaving and educational—*Why Me?*—was shown when most people were in bed.

"My biggest objection to *Why Me?* was the coding we have on TV, relating to the bare breast. [The program] was shown too late at night. I take my children to the Slurpee machine and here is *Cosmopolitan* with some girl's crotch hanging over the Slurpee machine, and I go, *Well, now where are our values?* Somehow there is something wrong somewhere. [By now, we are all laughing in agreement.]

"We are all so complex. It must be incredibly hard to try to reach all women. I admire you for taking a stab at it. I had a lot of prior knowledge, so we could handle our situation and work with it. But as young women, let us begin to educate our young daughters and sons to these things.

"How lucky we are to be living now when there are things that can be done. In the past, women at thirty had eight or nine kids, were falling apart at the seams, and were either very old women at forty, or dead. I consider myself eligible to wear pigtails and silk ribbons until I am fifty."

"A mother's love endures through all. . . . She remembers the infant smiles that once filled her bosom with rapture, the merry laugh, the joyful shout of his childhood, the opening promise of his youth. . . ."
—Washington Irving
American author (1783–1859)

"Look at a man in the midst of doubt and danger, and you will learn in his hour of adversity what he really is. It is then that true utterances are wrung from the recesses of his breasts. The mask is torn off, the reality remains."

—LUCRETIUS
Roman poet (circa 99–55 B.C.)

7

HUSBAND REACTIONS

"I will fasten on this sleeve of thine:
Thou are an elm, my husband, I, a vine."
—William Shakespeare
English playwright and poet (1564–1616)

"CLINICAL WORK AND RESEARCH STUDIES HAVE SHOWN that cancer does indeed invade the entire family, and that family members, especially spouses, are often highly distressed individuals. The family in general and the spouse in particular cannot, therefore, be looked on as natural supporters for cancer patients, but rather as a system that is itself in need of help and support."[1]

Cancer is a family crisis, and as women who have undergone the mastectomy, we must set the tone for acceptance. If we are unable to do this, how can we expect our husbands to do so, particularly when they are also emotionally distressed?

Before she died several months after our interview, Janice (39/39) expressed her concern that there is no program to help the husbands like the American Cancer Society has for females. "He should be able to cry and talk to somebody about this," she said.

Some women feel they have completely accepted their mastectomy, but their words reflect otherwise. Jessie (46/46) belligerently stated, "You must have a hang-up to write this book." There was no peace in her behavior, and this negatively affected her family.

Committed marriages—built on friendship, love, trust, and respect—survive the loss of breasts. These husbands and wives bond even closer, often attaining a deeper devotion, understanding, and tenderness toward each other. The majority of the seventy women had such marriages and accepted our mastectomies, knowing our husbands to be pillars of strength, love, and devotion. They became giants in our eyes.

Women in troubled marriages often blamed failure on the mastectomy, while later admitting there were many prior problems that led to the breakdown of their relationships. Troubled marriages either continue in their misery, or dissolve in divorce courts where the mastectomy and the "womanizer" are the accused. Laura (58/65) felt that her husband "could have cared less... It would have been a way out for him, as he was seeing another woman. He did tell our children he would come back to take care of me and he did for one month." They later divorced.

Our Experiences in Troubled Marriages

Blanche (47/48), married 26 years: "He can't face problems."

"My husband acted nonchalant. I have a few problems with him. He can't face problems. Something comes up, and it really bothers him. I said how ugly it looked, and he said, 'No, it does not look bad at all.' This is really all the discussion we had. There are several problems. I'm having some problems in my marriage and am not having as nice a sex life. Sex has never been that big to me, and it hasn't bothered my husband."

Joleen (38/41), married four years: "I probably drove him further away from me."

"This is my second marriage and the mastectomy has most certainly affected my sexual life in sundry ways. A lot of it has to do with my personality and my husband's personality—the foundation upon which we had our relationship of a marriage. I frequently wonder just what was the most influential part of it as far as our association, whether his reaction was the bad one or mine was the bad one. I don't really know. A year and a half later, we did go our separate ways. I'm sure the mastectomy contributed a great deal to our parting. We separated for three months, then reestablished ourselves on solid ground, and came back together.

"The mastectomy had a good influence and a bad influence. He was a womanizer, and I knew this when I married him. I married him, knowing full well what the circumstances were and was prepared to deal with it. I was a busy executive, and he had his law practice. We each had our own lives, and it was nice to be married, but it was more superficial than it is now. After my mastectomy, as much as I tried to rationalize that I could react badly to him as a result of it, I couldn't control the fact that I probably did. I probably drove him further away from me.

"My husband saw the scar at home and was putting on a very brave front for me. Normally he wasn't reviled by anything. It was a blow to him. It wasn't until after I left him and came back to him that we really discussed the emotional impact of it on him. I said, 'It has been two-and-a-half years since my mastectomy. How did you really feel?' He said he felt cheated. I said, 'OK, I can accept that. Now tell me why you felt cheated.' He answered, 'Because you did have a beautiful body.'

"We would go to Las Vegas together, and I would wear low-cut gowns, and he took personal pride in walking through a casino where other people turned around to look at me. He had been the envy of many men as a result of my figure. It is rather ridiculous and childish, but nevertheless, it is a matter of fact. Since we were initially attracted to each other because of our physical attraction to one another, it is reasonable that he should have felt cheated. When we discovered that we had more together than the physical, we could discuss it. He had less and less interest in me sexually. I felt this, and there was little I could do. I felt helpless. I wasn't sure that I wasn't acting in a way that was driving him away, so it was a frustration. I can never be sure if I was driving him away.

"I can see from other people's circumstances that very subtle things can take place, and frequently the obvious is not the matter of fact. So I do search my own feelings and reactions. Sexually I felt awkward, very awkward. He tried so hard not to be, but we both felt awkward. It is no longer of any consequence.

"My husband was of course trying to protect me. He was telling me that it was of no consequence, he loved me and not the breast. It was a case of us both, more or less protecting each other. Very intriguing and intricate thing, this husband-and-wife situation. I left my husband."

Our Experiences with Committed Marriages

Alice (39/47): "Now sexually I'm not satisfied."

"This is my second marriage. All women are scared of what their husbands feel. I just took his word that it didn't make any difference. There were no sexual changes. I told the doctor that now sexually I'm not satisfied, and my husband's not satisfied. He said the chemotherapy is drying you up, use Vaseline. I can't climax anymore; I'm so dry down there. The doctor said to send in my husband and he would talk to him. I just don't have the desire and haven't for almost four years."

Kitty (29/31): "My husband has just been marvelous."

"A wonderful thing happened. I met my second husband in January 1973, and we were married in June. My mastectomy had been in November of the previous year. He is fantastic. When I am down, he will not let me be defeated. Initially, I felt apprehensive about sex, but because of the attitude of my husband, he assured me right away, there was no problem. He said it made absolutely no difference, so it made no difference. I felt very fortunate that way. I have noticed a lessening in sexual desire on my part since I have been on chemotherapy. I'm just not as eager as I used to be for sex. I haven't asked the doctor; maybe I should. My husband has just been marvelous. I really lucked out."

Denise (56/57), married 38 years: "I looked at his face and he accepted it."

"My husband has accepted it very well. He is very kind and is accepting it beautifully. There are no sex problems as a result of surgery. I was afraid to show him my scar, but he was very kind and nice. I looked at his face and he accepted it. That made me feel much better. I had seen the scar when they dressed it. I felt I had to live with it, so I made up my mind and have accepted it all right. I've just got to do it—use faith."

Donna (41/42), married 23 years: "We don't shower together anymore."

"I don't keep my bra on, but intercourse is in the dark. Naturally you think it would affect our sex life if I won't even look at the scar myself or show it to him, but it hasn't. The only way it has affected us is that we don't shower together anymore. We don't do that kind of thing anymore. There is no daytime sex. I don't want him to see, and I don't think it is necessary for him to see. Oh, no, I would never even let other women see me. Whenever I get out of the shower, I just drape the towel over me as I stand in front of the mirror. I can't believe any woman who says it is not important to have a breast there. How do you feel about yours? Evidently you feel better about yours than I do. It is the look in your eye that says you don't understand what I am saying.

"My husband is a neat guy and says it doesn't matter. I've told him how I feel. He said I'm better than a lot of women with two breasts. He says all the right things, and I would like to believe him, but that is hard to believe. I know that we get along good. I guess it is vanity, I'm sure it is vanity. I think every day is a gift, and I had better live it fully."

Jennifer (27/27), married five years: "He just hugged me."

"Sex is probably even better because we have been through so much lately. My husband is beautiful. When showing my scar to my husband, I said, 'It is going to be horrible and going to be ugly,' and he just hugged me and said it was going to be OK. I said, 'Are you prepared for this?' It was something I wanted to get over with right away. He said, 'You are the one with the problem, because you have to learn to live with this for the next fifty years.' He accepts it, but I have trouble accepting, because I don't have a breast; so it is my problem and not his. I guess I am really vain. It doesn't bother me when I walk around during the day, but when I look in the mirror, I feel kind of—it is a dumb word—but kind of *deformed* in a horrible sort of way. Kind of deformed."

Opal (34/56), married thirty-five years: "My husband was just concerned about my life."

"The breast—so what? A lot of people lose an arm or a leg, and both of us felt this way. I was small, about 110 pounds, and both of us just felt good. There is no way people without an arm or leg can hide this disfigurement. I was small busted, and it wouldn't show that much. There were no problems sexually, not at all."

Tressa (33/33), newly wed: Fiancé said, "I understand and it doesn't matter."

"I knew through this whole thing that there was someone there that loved me no matter what, my fiancé. He would love me without breasts as I would love him without arms. I felt that strongly about it. I had that feeling night and day. Through the whole thing, we decided not to wait another six months to decide when to get married. We decided to do it now, at a time when it would be beneficial to me about not having to go back to work to support my two children from a previous marriage. He also has two children from a previous marriage. Even so, I knew I could never let him look at me, which is not true.

"My fiancé came into the bathroom. I covered myself and walked out of the bathroom and went to pieces. He cried with me and said, 'I understand, and it doesn't matter.' I said, 'I can never let you see me, I can *never* let you see me.' He said, 'Yes, you will, and it will be all right.' When I had to change the bandage and couldn't use my arm and became frustrated, he asked, 'Can I help you?' I said yes. I thought that this is the man I love and he loves me and this is something I have to do. Even though I don't want him to see it, that is my pride, but I knew he will still love me. So I had to make that choice. He was so good. He put his arms around me and said, " Honey, I know why you feel so bad, but it is not that bad.' And I said, 'Ah, that was so easy.' The thought was worse than the reality. We were married in October 1974."

Robin (60/62), married seventeen years: "Nothing bothers him. I came first."

"My husband is a merchant marine. I have an unusual husband, but I feel you should talk everything over with each other. Nothing bothers him. I came first. He didn't care if I was all carved up; I came first. I was alive, and he still says that. My husband is fourteen years younger than me, and it took him two years to convince me that age didn't make a difference. So I married him."

Nan (55/59), married thirty-nine years: "We have faith in God."

"My husband has dressed the scar. He is more concerned about me as a person, as his wife. My husband is sorry, but he is not the type of person to be upset about that alone. My family is raised with sons [ages] thirty-one and thirty-six. We have faith in God."

Margaret (48/49), married sixteen years: Husband said, "I didn't marry you for your breast."

"I called my husband and told him not to bother to come to the hospital, because we were all through—finished—and I would never feel the same, that I wouldn't want him to live with me. And, oh, it was just terrible. It really hit me very hard. He tried to reassure me that it didn't make any difference at all, but I said no, that we had talked about this before, and that we were finished. When I went home, I looked around and nothing had changed. The kids were there and the dogs were there, the clock, but everything had changed in my life. I had the tendency to lock myself up in my bedroom and just cry. Little by little you come to grips with this. My husband said he would like to quietly go away and have a nervous breakdown. But he is a very strong person and really is my pillar of strength.

"My husband said, 'That is a beautiful scar. It is there. It doesn't make any difference. I didn't marry you for your breasts to begin with. I don't want you to go into hiding; I don't want you to turn out lights.' Without my family encouraging me, I never could have done it.

"To be honest about sex, in my case it did make a difference, because I was used to very low nightgowns. I had beautiful breasts, which were my pride, and all my gowns were sexy. That was all over. It didn't make any difference to my husband, but I definitely felt a diminished interest. I always had low clothes to show off my breasts because they were my best feature. I really mourned the loss of my breast until I found out about my other cancer problems. It is my life I'm fighting for now. The breast is not that important."

Grace (46/57), married thirty-three years: "He is very sensitive and tender."

"My husband is a very hard-working, dear man, a tremendous help. I didn't let my husband see the scar for a long time, not because of any fear on my part that he would no longer like me or love me, but even minor injuries bothered him. Being involved in the medical profession is the last thing he would want to do. He is very sensitive and tender. I didn't see any point in him seeing it. When he did see it, his reaction was that it was tragic, but that thank goodness, we had hopefully caught it in time. This has made absolutely no difference sexually."

Becky (51/51), married thirty-one years: "It was not the loss of the breast, but that he might lose me."

"My poor husband, the best husband in the world. He is the Rock of Gibraltar for his entire family. He just blocked cancer out completely. He just couldn't believe that this could happen to me. He was sick, sick, sick, not because I was going to be disfigured or any dumb thing like that, but because there was a chance of losing me. It was not the loss of the breast, but that he might lose me.

"If anything, at our age—he being sixty and I am fifty-one—at this point it even brought a new tenderness into our sex relationship, based upon the fact that some of our embraces had to be changed. My husband has been wonderfully considerate in making these adjustments, and doing it without making me aware that he is doing it. So our relationship is closer sexually perhaps more than it has ever been."

Della (47/52), married thirty-two years: "I can lean on him."

"My husband saw the scar and didn't act any way but accepting of it. My husband is a stable person and very unemotional outwardly, but emotional inwardly. He would also put on the best front possible, because he is always supportive of me. I can lean on him. He teaches business education in a high school. Sexually, my husband has never made me feel anything less than what I was before."

Beatrice (54/55), married five years: "My husband loves me."

"My friends told me that my husband was really shook about cancer, but he didn't say anything to me. I don't think this makes any difference to my husband, because he loves me. However, I would never dream of letting him see me. So help me God, he is never going to see. I can hardly stand it myself."

Andrea (39/43), married twenty-two years: "My husband was very calming and kind."

"I can remember saying to him two months earlier that I could stand just about anything except losing a breast. I never knew anyone with a mastectomy, even though I had two years of nurse's training. I will never forget his reaction either: 'Honey, if something like that ever happened, it would be just one of those things; I wouldn't love you any less, because you wouldn't be a different person. And should it happen, think of it as just one more hurdle we go through.'

"He had a great deal of gentleness and concern for my feelings. He never said those words, but that is the message he tried to convey. Always a great deal of support. My husband saw the scar when he helped me change the bandage. I told him I could do it, but would he like to, and he said yes. I cried the whole time, because I didn't want him to see it. He acted in a very professional manner, which was probably the very best thing for me, objective until after he had the dressing changed. Then we both just dissolved into tears together. That was good.

"Our sex life has not changed, afraid not. [She laughed.] The concern I had at first was wondering what was he thinking. In a way, that was unfair to him after being married to him as long as I have. He probably wasn't thinking much differently than he always thought during an occasion like that. I was reserved. A couple years before the mastectomy, I was getting to feel pretty good about my body and would go through the game of putting on a gown and the fun of ripping it off, and all that. Well, I did not do that now, and he never asked me if I wanted to take my gown off. I think he instinctively understood that if the time ever came when I wanted to, I would do it. Which I did, eventually.

"When I was undergoing radiation, I became extremely tired. My husband was very understanding. So there was a gap there where I had very little interest in sex. I never bared myself in front of him completely nude. I assumed he had not seen the scar again until this warm night in San Jose. I said, 'This nightgown is really hot,' and he said, 'Why don't you do what you usually do when you are hot.' I said, 'Well, I will take it off,' and he said, 'Why don't you?' And I did, and I can remember very specifically watching his face. I know that was stupid, but I did, and his expression never changed, and I thought, *Well, I'm home free.* Which I knew all along, but I needed the reassurance."

Esther (44/57), married thirty-six years: "I don't like to see a man cry."

"My husband was concerned over me, and he has a beautiful attitude about it. He thinks it is ridiculous for men to take an attitude about the loss of a breast. He said, 'What is the difference? I have one kidney.' My husband is overly sentimental. He cried when he saw the scar. It made me feel bad, because I don't like to see a man cry."

Bertha (64/64), married forty-three years: "He said it was not ugly to him."

"One day, for some reason, I was facing my husband without a brassiere and I said, 'Oh, honey, I know this must be ugly.' He said, it was not ugly to him, and that was the kindest thing in the world. He said, 'I suppose it is ugly as far as scars go, but it doesn't bother me.'"

Heather (64-65/66), married forty-five years: "He said if it has to be, it has to be."

"He has been wonderful through the whole thing. I [wondered] how could my husband bear to look at me like that? He has always been *very* supportive and loving and tender. It was so ugly. He said that I still have buttocks and legs. His attitude from the very beginning was, what if it had been an arm or a leg? This has helped me a great deal."

Judy (51/53), married thirty-six years: "I didn't marry you for them."

"My husband said, 'After all, I didn't marry you for any part of your body in particular, I didn't marry you for breasts.' He has been very good about that and said he doesn't have to look at the scar. I go without my bra in front of my children, but fully dressed."

Daisy (59/62), married twelve years: "He died five months ago."

"My husband was very distressed, for just six months prior to my operation, he had a commando operation of the mouth for cancer. He was upset for me, not himself. He was a very emotional person anyway. I was distressed about sex with my husband at first, and thought that maybe it would make a difference, and was building this in my mind. But it didn't make any difference. He tried very hard to reassure me and said there was no reason for me to be worried. He said, 'It doesn't bother me, therefore don't let it bother you.' I believed him. He died five months ago."

Jan (32/32), married thirteen years: "He is a wonderful guy, an inspiration."

"My husband was stunned. He loses his patience with me at times. I know my attitude can affect them all. Sometimes I get so low and down that I don't believe anybody, but he is a wonderful guy, an inspiration."

Rose (49/49), married thirteen years: "He wanted to share the worry."

"As a nurse, you felt the doctor's word was law. My husband was very angry that I didn't tell him about the lump. I wanted to protect him, but he wanted to share the worry. He has been very good and said that the scar is not bad at all. As for sex, I was reticent at first, but as long as it doesn't bother him, I have to live with it."

Glenda (55/55), married thirty-four years: "The very best has come out of him."

"As for my husband, there has been beautiful acceptance. It has only been two weeks since surgery and my husband just keeps saying, hurry up and feel better. He is a very sweet person. My first concern was that I said I didn't expect to look like a little monster. I was teasing him by saying, you are now to go out and find yourself a pretty little chick. He got very upset and said, 'I love *you*.'

"That is just what I needed to hear, of course. I said it because I wanted him to feel free. I wanted a free choice. I didn't want him to feel that he was held to anything. Whatever his reaction was, I wanted it to come from within himself. Does that sound strange? You would have to know me as a person, because I feel that one has to be free. You cannot make a person feel obligated or feel you have to lean on him to hold him in any way. We have been married for thirty-four years. I don't care how long you are married, you are not sure of what his reaction will be. You never really know until you face this.

"It is not the breast; isn't that strange? Maybe it is because we are rather proud of our bodies. At least I have always tried to maintain myself and to be a whole person. All of a sudden, I felt I am not a whole person. Strangely enough, now I don't even think about it until I look into a mirror, and then I think, *How strange.* I don't seem to care. My own feelings don't seem to be involved.

"It makes no difference to him. He is pretty honest, and I would know by his attitude, because I know him so well. The strange thing is, believe it or not, what is inside of a person comes out at a time like this, and the very best has come out of him. He is kinder and more loving than he has ever been, and I don't think it is pity. Something has awakened from his inner self, because it really does bring out the truth in a person."

Marie (42/42) married six years (now thirty-one years): His honesty was comforting.

When I was told that I needed surgery for possible cancer, I never asked, 'Why me?' That question would imply that cancer should have happened to someone else. I cried because of overwhelming sadness at the possibility that death would take me away from my beloved husband.

My mother tenderly helped me bathe my wound at home, and I planned to wait for further healing before showing Bill the scar, as he had no experience with surgery. Sudden, unexpected muscle spasms began in my chest wall and frightened me, because the doctor had not explained this possibility. Difficulty finding a comfortable sleeping position and continued spasms left me exhausted: both led to a delay in exposing my chest to my husband.

One evening, I asked Bill if he felt prepared to look at my scar, and he said, "Yes, I always have been ready." We went into my bathroom. I slowly removed the bandage and kept my eyes on his face, while asking him if he thought the scar was ugly. What a relief when he honestly said, "Yes, but I don't think any scar is pretty." All tension left me as I knew he was speaking only of my wound, not of me. Our sex life continued to be filled with tender consideration for each other.

Interviews with Four Husbands

Hal: married to Ethel (41/47) for twenty-six years.

"I knew before the surgery that it was cancer, but she didn't. I knew the night before, because the doctor told me. I didn't want to tell her because she was in such a good frame of mind. I did not want to put anything in her mind or change her frame of mind. I thought I would just leave things alone, since she was facing things just fine. I knew what had to be done, that it would have to be a radical mastectomy. I was impressed just knowing what was going to happen, you know, complete removal of the breast. I was wondering what her feelings would be if I told her, because I don't think she had anything serious on her mind when she went to the hospital.

"I didn't have any particular feeling when I heard about it at first because it seemed so far-removed. I was just surprised at the scar; it was so neat. I was surprised that the nipple was gone. I thought there might be some semblance of a nipple left. No, just diagonal, *zoom*, everything was gone. There were no sexual problems [both agreed]. A breast is like a trimming on a cake. If the trimming is gone, the cake is still there."

Kent: husband of Beth (40/51) who died ten days before our planned interview.

"Women need to talk about this; they need the ability to talk. Guys will react in different ways: they will either walk away, ignore it, or live with it. You never know what a person will do under stress. It depends upon how selfish you are, how concerned, and how important family relationships are to you. You would be surprised at the way people act. The philanderer who always fights with his wife comes through like a trooper, while the devoted husband goes off the deep end. One man in the hospital cried and asked, 'Why me?' and I thought, *Hell, she is the one being all cut up and who will be in pain and have to live with it*. But he felt, *Why me?*

"You can't say anything to men. By the time it happens, they will be in their middle ages and will do what they will do. It is something that unfolds; it is just like lightening striking you. The first time we were told Beth would not live, we were brave and all that, and then nine months later she was working. We said, didn't we act like pure fools?

"Beth fought a brilliant delaying action. Expect a miracle, and she did expect a miracle. She lived eleven-and-a-half years longer than expected. Our daughters have been real Trojans."

Merv (50): business associate of my husband.

"My wife had surgery sixteen years ago, radical of the right breast. She was reticent about sex, but I didn't care. I continued to act as I did before and caressed her as though she had a breast. Older men are more mature and realize there is more to a relationship than breasts. Greatest fear is of recurrence, not of losing the other breast, but of losing my wife. Younger men place more emphasis on the body. The scar is not pretty. We have a long-standing, permanent relationship. There should be complete truth between partners."

Bill (46): my husband.

"I was shocked. I was concerned for you and I remember you crying. When we first met the surgeon, Dr. S., he was calm, cool, collected, and positive. Seemed to be very confident in his own ability, and he was soothing. He gave us both confidence.

"The first day was the hardest, but after your mother came, you were very calm. Your mom asked about how you were taking it, and I tried to reassure her. I felt sorry for you, not knowing how extensive it was. It was a feeling for you. No, I wasn't concerned about losing the breast, I was concerned about losing everything, of losing you.

"It was a long wait while you were in surgery. We were hoping that you would come out in a couple of hours and say that it was not malignant. The doctor was delayed in going into your operation. I think you went in at 10 A.M., and the doctor didn't come out until about 3:30 P.M. He said he had to remove the breast, and as far as he could tell, he got everything. We were relieved.

"I took a week off work for the surgery. I think I talked to some friend but don't remember. I first saw you in the room after the recovery room, but you were pretty well out of it. You recognized me, and that was about it. I was the only one there. Your mother was concerned about feeding us at home, and everybody was so relieved that it was over. Your attitude in the hospital was very good. You were undoubtedly in a lot of pain for the first few days, but I thought your attitude was very good, and it was good at home.

"I had never seen a mastectomy scar before, but I could imagine what it would look like. I didn't think it would be so red and painful looking but it was what I expected and didn't expect anything different. When you asked me if I thought the scar was ugly, I said, 'Yes, but I don't think any scar is pretty.' I don't think a scar on your leg, arm, or any cut in the body is pretty. I wanted to see it, maybe curiosity, but I wanted to know what you had to put up with, and think you should show it. A husband should know what it looks like. It would be hiding something from someone when your not sharing. You should share.

"No, if you lost your other breast it would not be a catastrophe as far as I am concerned. It might be as far as you are concerned. I think it is better to do that than to lose your life. A scar is something that would not normally be there. It is like I would cut a hole in this table and it was not normally there; it is something different. You wouldn't deliberately make it that way. I think movies, magazines, and beauty contests place more emphasis on breasts than men, per se. It is the individual man. As far as I'm concerned, breasts are not that important. If I'm not mature now at my age, honey, I never will be.

"You ask how I might feel if I were single. I don't really know; it is hard to relate. I don't think it would make much difference if you are really fond of a person. People marry people who are blind, in wheel chairs. It depends upon what your relationship was before. If it is a casual relationship and you are not really serious about the person, it might make a difference if you had to weigh all factors as to which one of several women you were going to continue dating.

"If a man doesn't want a woman because she has lost a breast or both breasts, she ought to look somewhere else, if that is all that interests him. It wouldn't be a very lasting relationship, and she should say, 'Here's the door.'

"I would assure male friends that it is not the end of the earth; it is something that had to be removed to rid the body of cancer. It is no more than removing a finger or a big toe. Would you rather have a breast removed or your nose or your ear? I'm giving you alternatives to think about.

"You tell me that the women you are interviewing are handling themselves well, for the most part, but it is when they are in relationships with men that they are terribly upset. Maybe women place more emphasis on the breast than men do, or they think it is more important. I want you to be normal. You never ran around without a bra before, so why would you do it now? Be comfortable, be yourself.

"I can see that some women, who maybe don't have any smarts, feel that all they really have going for them is their body, think nobody will ever love them again if this happens to them, their husbands will leave them, etc. And they have no self-confidence—I can see that they will be devastated for years or a lifetime. Whereas, I think that you have self-confidence because loss of a breast is not the most important thing to you. Life is more important to you. Now, writing this book is the most important thing, because you hope to convince other women that a mastectomy is not the end of the earth. You have a good self-image, and your confidence will continue to carry you through. I love you."

"There is a peculiar beauty about godly old age—the beauty of holiness. Husband and wife who have fought the world side by side, who have made common stock of joy or sorrow, and become aged together, are not unfrequently found curiously alike in personal appearance, in pitch and tone of voice, just as twin pebbles on the beach, exposed to the same tidal influences, are each other's alter ego."

—Alexander Smith
Scottish poet (1830–1867)

"So ought men to love their wives as their own bodies. He that loveth his wife loveth himself . . . and the wife see that she reverence her husband."

—Ephesians 5:28, 33

"Beloved, let us love one another: for love is of God; and every one that loveth is born of God, and knoweth God. He that loveth not knowth not God; for God is love."

—1 John 4:7–8

"No coward soul is mine,
No trembler in the world's storm-troubled
    sphere:
I see Heaven's glories shine,
And faith shines equal, arming me from fear."

—EMILY BRONTË
English novelist (1818–1848)

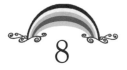

8

ACCEPTANCE AND ADJUSTMENT

"No one can make you feel inferior without your permission."

—*Eleanor Roosevelt*
Wife of Franklin Delano Roosevelt (1884–1962)

EACH WOMAN IS DIVINELY UNIQUE and grieves as an individual, not as a group. She grieves the loss of her breast and makes no apology as she struggles to understand feelings and emotions concerning her changed body image. Acceptance of this disfigurement is an incremental process, not an immediate once-and-for-all response. There are no absolutes on how to cope, just different paths to healing our hurts in order to adjust.

During the period of adjustment, some women are very private, while others crave human company. The seesaw emotions common to us all include: fear of recurrence and death, self-consciousness, apprehension over male acceptance or rejection, concern for our family, and problems with prosthesis and clothing. Bouts of depression and anger often occur, but they are the companions of cancer, and we fight them as courageously as we fight cancer.

Women with positive self-esteem see themselves as hopeful fighters, filled with faith in God, and determined not to give up. They speak of the loving support of their husbands, parents, friends, families, and colleagues. Daily, they deliberately strive to direct their minds toward productive thoughts and expectations. They value and appreciate life and want to make the most of every day, not just for themselves and their families, but also for the stranger in their midst. They choose life amidst tragedy—life filled with humor, purpose, and hope.

Women with negative self-esteem speak of self-pity, vanity, hatred of their changed body, escapism, and avoidance of social contact. They often dwell on what they can no longer do, instead of concentrating on what they can still do. New possibilities are foreign to their thinking. Dwelling in the past and second-guessing their medical treatment brings them hours of mental distress.

Our Experiences Dealing with Acceptance and Adjustment

Bernice (43/44): "A lot of prayers came my way and I think guided me."

"There were a lot of visitors while I was in the hospital. I wanted people. I didn't think of needing people at the time, but now that I look back on it, yes, I guess I needed people. I needed the attention. It made me feel that a heck of a lot of people cared about me. I didn't feel they did before. Maybe it is because I did not like myself before.

"Even now—a year and a half later—I still get tired, but I never had the stamina to keep going and going. Now I tire just that much sooner. I've learned to pace myself instead of push myself. My dad and his wife and a lot of friends helped me. But as my parents got ready to leave, I could feel the lump in my throat. I hoped and prayed that they would get out the door before I let it out, but I let it all out. Boy, I let go, and that delayed their leaving for about a half hour. It was just that they were neat about coming here and standing by; it was more their being such great parents. I was crying about that more than about the surgery.

"I went back to work on a half-day basis for one week, three weeks after surgery. Then I went back full time. My colleagues were curious, and I could feel them looking at my breasts, so I looked right back. They were trying to determine which one it was, and I wasn't going to tell them. Pretty soon they quit. Some of them didn't really think I had a mastectomy, because I think I acted just as normally as before. I would talk about it freely, sometimes maybe too much, but I would bring up the subject freely.

"People were not afraid then to ask questions, as I wasn't afraid to talk about it. I talked more than they asked questions. I need to talk about it, and they may have been afraid then to ask me questions because they weren't sure how I would react. But after I got it all talked out, they felt free to ask questions. One girl, whose mother found a lump in her breast, wanted me to talk to her. Yes, men wanted to talk, and that surprised me. One married man talked to me in depth about it. He was curious about it. I just didn't think that men at work would do that, personal friends, yes. I guess I was a victim of cancer. I was a mastectomy patient.

"I take articles on cancer with a grain of salt because a lot of them are not necessarily true, accurate. People bring articles in, saying that maybe breast cancer had a better cure than removing the breast. I say, 'Hey, that is fine, but that is in the future as far as I am concerned.' At the time my breast was removed, that was the only way that anyone knew how to do it. If things change, fine. Look at the people who were stricken with polio. Now that is changed, but this is part of our medical growing. I don't feel badly about having new ideas come up. I am more aware of cancer. If I get cancer again, it will be taken care of again; that is my reaction. It is not going to get me. There will be some way of taking care of me.

"What helped me the most to adjust to this surgery? That's a big question. Both my surgeon and family doctor are gentle and easy-going men. Their nonchalance about the whole thing kept me from becoming uptight. Perhaps my not questioning and not knowing protected me. Since I didn't know some of the ramifications of things, maybe it was easier for me to accept. Being a person that will go on blind faith, you might say, this could be good or this could be bad for me to tell anyone else. I'm just not the kind of person that will go out and look around. I'm not familiar with medicine and don't know how to suggest finding a doctor.

"Women react to the removal of a breast so strongly because it is part of their sexuality, I guess. But maybe this is an old wives' tale because most of the women I have talked to aren't all that concerned over the removal of the breast. Everyone is tip-toe-ing around saying, 'Oh, poor thing—*tsk, tsk,*—treat them gently.' I think this is hogwash. I haven't seen that many people saying, 'Poor me.' Most of them are saying, 'What's the difference, here?'

"I had to have some good strokes as I was afraid and self-conscious after my surgery. I knew I could handle it all right, but I didn't know if I was ready for a rejection because I was missing a breast. Maybe [I was] overly anxious to tell a man I was dating that I was minus a breast because they couldn't tell just by looking. Most of the men have been respectfully curi-ous. Is that a good term? They want to know all about it. Some of them ask questions right away, some later, some ignore it. But I can take the risk now.

"I work with Reach to Recovery and it is very rewarding. Most of the women are very positive, which surprised me. It is nice to talk to someone positive. I know they have their depres-sions. One of my friends who died of breast cancer had such a fantastic attitude. She said, 'I've had just this much more time with my kids.' This is what I keep running into and these mar-velous attitudes help build me up.

"I think that losing your other breast might be OK because I can't get things to fit me now, and I could be a size smaller. In the back of my mind, I think, *If the other one goes, does this mean I will have cancer other places? Will I be prone to cancer?* I push this away by thinking of all the lovely things I could get into if I were a B cup instead of a D cup.

"I was really depressed initially but I started to think, *Here I am a single lady, and I would like to marry again, and I don't know now if I could handle that or if anyone else could handle that.* I would have to wait to see. But my depression is something I have lived with for a long time. I became depressed not just over breast surgery but over my life. In fact, I am less depressed about my breast surgery than I was before. I've come to know myself a little better. I like myself a lot better. I think I had to begin to learn to like myself. I think it was about time. Something had to jar me into liking me, and I think the mastectomy has. A lot of prayers came my way, and I think they guided me.

"I had a friend-lover. He accepted me for what I was before and what I was after. We are good friends. He cares enough about me that he can be honest. I did a lot of joking about my surgery. He would say 'Don't do that; it puts you down.' I guess I joked because I wanted it out in the open. It was a cover, perhaps. I do it now sometimes when I feel ill-at-ease with people. I don't know why I do that.

"I told those men I thought I would get involved with that I had a prosthesis, [thinking], *Oh, wow, I better tell them so I won't get hurt. That's bad, hurt me! Tsk, tsk.* I don't want to be hurt. Now I would be able to risk a relationship more because I can say the mastectomy was not my doing. The fellow I'm dating now is moving to Arizona for a business opportunity. So OK, I've met a lot of people, so he leaves. There is a plan going on for me and for him. He may move back here, but there is something that is going to happen."

Alice (39/47): "Take each day as it comes."

"I am not cured, but the cancer is arrested under chemotherapy. When I had my ovaries and adrenal glands removed, a pastor of that hospital came in and said a prayer for me. He said, 'Undoubtedly you are needed in another world.' 'Oh God,' I said, 'I don't want to go; I've got kids, my kids need me.' He came back to apologize. I told my husband, 'Don't have that man come in to see me again, I think I'm going to die.'

"The women I know now that have a mastectomy are not sad or depressed and take each day as it comes—all except the younger girls who seem to have more problems, in their twenties. There was a girl twenty-six years old having her second breast removed and I went to talk to her.

"I broke down crying in front of you for the first time in eight years. I don't know, I felt sorry for myself at that time. I say it is because I had nobody around here to talk to me. Women would come to my door to see me, but I wouldn't answer the door because I didn't want anyone to see me like this. I don't like to break down in front of other people; it doesn't help other people."

Sarah (44/44): "It is easier for me if people just come up and talk to me about it."

"When I got home, I was bothered that the boys were always doing something. I wanted somebody around. That is the hardest part, because you have a lot of attention while you are in the hospital. I'm grateful to be alive, but I'm not sure if I had that choice again if I would go through that again. The pain. If I had to lose the second breast, it would be equally as hard, because this time I would be aware of the cancer and not the cosmetic.

"The first day back to work was probably the worst day. Oh, it was difficult. I was terribly self-conscious, thinking that everyone was staring at me and wondering which side it was. I would catch people looking at me and trying not to be obvious about it. There is one gal that has not spoken to me yet. She just can't talk to me, just turns her head every time I come near. I figure she has a worse problem than I have. I've tried to understand it but I don't. It is extremely difficult for her to talk to me at all. It is easier for me if people just come up and talk to me about it. I would rather they talk about it than sit and beat around the bush and forget that it happened, or pretend that it didn't happen."

Denise (56/57): "They do not come to our house anymore."

"All my people have accepted this, but not my husband's people. They will not visit our place anymore. They always tell my husband, 'Your wife is too sick.' I'm hurt, but I can understand because that is their way of life. His mother passed away from cancer of the female organs, a brother-in-law passed away from lung cancer, and they accepted both. But breast cancer is something else. They are afraid. I think they are afraid of the breast. My husband was in the medical corps when he was in the service. Naturally he is hurt that his family doesn't come, but they don't know any better. We have been married thirty-eight years. We have called and asked his sister and brother-in-law over, but they do not come to our house anymore."

Donna (41/42): "I can't wear a low-cut gown."

"My breasts are important to me, probably for a vain reason. When we grew up, it was fun to wear low-cut clothes and when

I got married, to dress up and to wear a bathing suit and go jump into the pool. These things I can't do and won't do anymore. I can't wear a low-cut gown.

"My breasts are also important because mostly it was important to my husband, and I knew that. He likes breasts. He thought that was pretty neat if you were well endowed and were able to show them off. A lot of men do. I know he has tried to convince me for a whole year, not that we talk about this because we don't. He has done everything imaginable to make me feel that I'm still just as neat as I always was, but underneath I can't feel that because I'm sure he is not telling the truth. Don't ask me why, because never once has he acted as though he were never telling the truth. You sense that because maybe I knew that it was important. I assumed it was important, but within twenty-three years of marriage, I guess you know it is important.

"I would not like to read a lot of stuff on cancer. I have a very low tolerance for pain and all that good stuff. I don't know how I raised four boys. How could I raise four boys with bleeding, etc.? Yes, childbirth was painful, but it is over, and you have a child. It is beautiful and does not relate or equate to the mastectomy at all. This is taking something away. I should have read more before the mastectomy. Statistics do bother me.

"I am living a normal life except within my own feeling. We still go dancing, but I can't wear the low dresses, and I don't like that. I tried wearing three of them, before giving them to my sister."

Jennifer (27/27): "My mother tried to keep me an invalid as long as she could."

"She stayed five days. How did my mother react? That is the hardest question of all to answer. Once she said she wished it was her. I don't know how she reacted. You have to know my mother. To give you an idea, she thinks I can plan for this next mastectomy and should hire a woman. So I don't want to talk about my mother [sighing], OK?

"I'm afraid of cancer. It did not go to my lymph nodes. I don't want to hear anything more unpleasant. I don't want to hear beyond right here and right now. I'll face it if it ever happens again."

Opal (34/56): "I had read the Bible and believed in God."

"If people have other emotional turmoil in their life, they can see the difference. Alcoholism was becoming a problem in our life and developed into a great emotional thing. If you ever live through that and make it through with sanity, you can appreciate the other things that come on. My husband is a recovered alcoholic, but for ten years he was pretty much out of control, and for five years it was quite an emotional thing. This is a bigger adjustment than losing a breast.

"Losing a breast may not cause one to seek a faith in a higher power, while there is nothing like alcoholism to cause one to do that. I had read the Bible and believed in God but didn't understand too much. But with alcoholism, I really sought to find a way to live my life in peace and comfort. The mastectomy has never been a major thing.

"At home after the mastectomy, I was not able to do much at first. As soon as I could get up and do my work, such as vacuum and straighten furniture, I then did an awful lot. I hung the clothes on the line, because I didn't have a dryer, so this helped me use my arm. It was really an achievement to hang the laundry.

"A year ago, I had open-heart surgery. You think you have problems with a mastectomy, try open-heart surgery. There is a world of difference. I don't think I would ever question the doctor's opinion. I would leave it up to the doctor. I told my doctor, 'Wait a minute, you are the doctor. God looks after both of us, and my faith has put me in His care and in yours: you take care of the mechanic part, and God will do the healing.'"

Tressa (33/33): "Positive thoughts, just feeling life."

"What helped me adjust? That is a good question. Two things. I have spent many hours alone with myself—and not locked up—reading and thinking, and just experiencing the moments as they go by because I thought, *I will never take this day for granted.* I'm just enjoying whatever I am doing. Positive thoughts, just feeling life. I've been divorced ten years. I don't know if spending time with myself would have been enough if my fiancé had not been there.

"The attitude of my doctor at first infuriated me because he was so casual, like he was going to take a splinter out of my finger.

This was his whole attitude. He was being casual with my body, and I really resented it. I wanted more concern, but when I got it, I didn't need it.

"I had people walking into my hospital room—very dear friends came in and fell apart—and I thought, *This I don't need.* They had come to cheer me up but instead sat by my bed and cried in the hospital. They asked, 'How can you sit there and not be upset?' I said, 'I am upset.' They were not hurting for me but for themselves, at how they would feel if it were them. They didn't realize that, and I did. They said, 'I came here and you make me feel strong because you are smiling.' I understood them. I said, 'Hey, look around you; there are a lot of things to smile about. If you want to look for the sad things, go ahead and look for them as they are there. It depends upon what you want.'

"I can look at my body and say it is not very nice, but it is all I've got. I can smile and even make jokes about it a bit, like the time I was gardening and both prosthesis fell on the ground. I have not overcome my disappointment at times and doubt that I ever will. I wish I had the breasts to offer my husband. Every once in a while I can feel, or think I feel, he was going to reach for this part of my body during intercourse. I asked him about it once, because I didn't know if I were projecting it or not. He said yes. That hurts. Even I feel sometimes my breast is itching [phantom pain] and then realize there is nothing there, and it is a disappointment. I liked my breasts—they were a part of me—like I like the rest of me, and I wish I had them back. I don't know if I will ever not say that."

Robin (60/62): *"So there is an organist without a falsie."*

"The hospital was a rest for me, a sojourn. I enjoyed it. Everyone was so kind. I faced it right away and looked at the scar in the mirror. I am an organist in the Elks Club. They all knew I have a mastectomy, but one night we had a big meeting and three presidents of the group were there. I was in a hurry to leave the house and never noticed a thing until I got up to play the organ and found I forgot the falsie.

"So there is an organist without a falsie. But the sash hid that, and afterward I thought, *I can't go anywhere like this,* and I started to stuff my bra with tissue. Someone saw me, and they fined me for forgetting my falsie—one of those fund fines. But I wasn't embarrassed and they weren't either, or they would not have dared to fine me publicly about it."

Vanessa (56/60): "I began a period of using terrible swear words."

"At home I was terribly tired and melancholia set it, but they had prepared my husband for that. My doctor told him there would be quite an adjustment, and you never knew when it was going to come. I began a period of using terrible swear words. I used to say *damn* or *hell*, but I went through this period. My nurse friend told me I was giving vent to my emotions in that way.

"I read everything about cancer, hoping there are more ways for detection and cures. I remember the surgeon said that sometimes they can save the nipple. I thought, *Why the heaven would you want the nipple on a flat piece of skin?* Maybe surgeons run out of things to say. I don't know [laughing].

"I did not tell my twenty-four-year-old son nor my baby brother. I didn't want them to worry. My son's friend kept him so busy, and that is what I wanted. I didn't want him to have time to think. I told him I had cancer, that I wasn't going to die, that they had to remove one of those funny little breasts, and that I would be tired for a long time. My husband is so perfect. I've read where men took it very, very hard and rejected the woman."

Nan (55/59): "I'm not one to give up."

"I have my head on straight. That helps to adjust. I have a nice family that has stood by me. I can have a lot of living to do yet. I'm not one to give up. You have your low points at times, but I have faith that I will come through. I will take one day at a time."

Ethel (41/47): "I am now a stronger human being."

"You can't really believe that it is happening to you. I was convinced that it had to be cancer because I couldn't see any reason for the nipple secretion color to be changing. It is a horrible word. You know, people are still scared of the word and what it means.

"I enjoyed my recovery because we had a housekeeper for the first three weeks, which I never had before, so I was living it up.

My anxieties were for my husband—just looking five years ahead, hoping there would be no recurrence or problems. At the time, we told the children that their mother lost a breast and that is about all.

"It wasn't like something you had to get fixed up, like a wooden arm. I never wore bikinis anyway, so it didn't make that much difference. That should be the least of anybody's worries; you should be concerned if you are going to recover. My scar is now a part of me. Time goes by, and you remain healthy. I know the first year I did not buy any new clothes because I thought, *I'm not going to waste his money.* Thoughts of death cross your mind. I'm not ready for death.

"I've often thought of having the other breast removed. With problems of prosthesis, it might be easier to have two instead of being lopsided. I would do it if necessary. I wouldn't be frightened this time, even knowing the implications.

"My thought was to protect my family and not cause them to think that I was devastated. [I wanted to] help them to recognize that it wasn't a problem that was going to take me away from them or anything. All the fears I felt, I had to hide from my children and husband. I had struggled to keep my husband and our marriage very, very happy, with no negatives. I never fought with him, I never argued with him, I was a very permissive wife. If I disagreed with something he did, I kept it to myself and dealt with it myself.

"I felt I had to carry this attitude through the mastectomy, and although I felt somewhat devastated, I felt I had to protect my husband from that. This is all fine, but eventually the piper has to be paid. So I have had emotional struggles myself. It was not the loss of the breast, but mortality that frustrated me the most. The physical part of it made me very, very sad. I had a relatively sedentary kind of job and could work and concentrate on other people's problems, thereby eliminating my tears and fears as much as possible.

"The removal of the second breast would not be as traumatic. I've come to terms with mortality. It is not the length of one's life as much as the quality. I can obliterate my chances of having a happy life by being full of fear. There is a supreme being and I've come to a nonstop conclusion that I need to examine why this has happened to me. Perhaps I can help someone else from dying of this disease by setting an example, if nothing else. Simply by surviving, living a satisfactory, fulfilled life.

"I'm a fairly level-headed woman, with a certain amount of reason and logic. I began taking sculpture lessons and have become an accomplished sculptor, and it was a diversion from my marriage. I resigned from the business and felt a need to express myself. I needed something to leave my children. I felt the urgency to learn as much and as quickly as I could. After leaving my husband, I became infatuated with a sculptor who helped me to learn that the breast was absolutely of no consequence to my sexual power. The loss of my breast couldn't have meant less to him, even as a sculptor that is so aware of the human form. His complete acceptance of me was so helpful.

"If the mastectomy has done anything for me, it has reassured me on the physical plane, certainly; and the sculptor has done a great amount for me in helping me establish my own self-esteem, because I do have an extraordinary talent, thus I am very, very fortunate. Artist work assures me that there will never be a time in my life that I will be bored, always something to learn, to do, exciting. I've been able to express myself and reveal myself more than ever in my life. I am a stronger human being."

Margaret (48/49): "I'm very hopeful. I have a strong faith."

"My breasts were always a great pride to me. I had a beautiful bustline. Some other women I knew had the mastectomy, and I told my husband that if that ever happened to me I would divorce him and not stay with him at all. When he came to the hospital, he said to stay calm and we will talk this over and it doesn't make any difference—the same things all husbands say.

"I was feeling reasonably well and even went to the hair dresser. We stopped for lunch. It is very difficult to describe my reaction. It is different, it fluctuates. My breasts were always a great pride to me. One day I am fine or I wake up in the middle of the night and have what they call 'terror in the night.' I have read a lot on chemotherapy and think it is a very hopeful field. I'm very hopeful. I have a strong faith."

Grace (46/57): "I am not in the least bit less feminine."

"I knew the loss of a breast would be a problem, as far as clothes were concerned. It has been and will always be. I didn't like that, but again felt fortunate that they caught it in time. I can't wear deep, narrow V-necklines. I'm not in the least bit less feminine. I might feel differently if I were single, but I don't really know. My husband has made me feel more cherished than ever.

"I'm a fighter and am opposed to the lack of medical schools and lack of doctors. This makes many doctors apparently overworked. Secondly, the impersonal attitude of many of the doctors."

Becky (51/51): "I want to live."

"There is an eight-year age difference between me and my husband, and we have an eight-year-old daughter, and he assumed that I would live forever. I have always been hale and hearty, never been medically ill in any sense of the word. I had all my parts, was fifty-one years old, and my husband had never anticipated that perhaps I might die before he did—except perhaps in an accident, but not from a medical reason. I understood his reaction because his concern was for his family, and he has always been great.

"I had already predetermined exactly what my philosophy would be should I be confronted with this disease. That is, I want to live a lot, and I will pay whatever price is necessary to pay for my life. If a little disfigurement, loss of tissue, can make me live another twenty years, they can have it. I thought the scar was beautiful and was very, very pleased. I expected it to be just like it was, great. I have seen many women with the Halsted method, which for a long time was all there was."

Blanche (47/48): "Everyone at work was so great."

"I wasn't used to having company, because when I went in for surgery, I never told anybody. I just didn't realize that many people cared. I thought that was the nicest thing I had ever had. Everyone at work was glad to see me back, were concerned that I didn't lift things, and hired two extra people to help me.

"There are clothing problems. My husband said, 'You never bothered about low-cut gowns before, why now?' I said that they never were in style before. I go out and buy a pattern and fabric, make it, and then it dawns on me, *How can I wear this open-backed dress?* I just couldn't figure out how to have the "backless" bra support it. So now the dress hangs in our closet with different kinds of styles. Maybe it is just that I want to wear this to show people there is nothing wrong with me, that I am still a woman. I don't know. I never really thought about it until my husband mentioned it.

"My eighty-two-year-old mother is almost blind and told my dad she wanted to see me before I died, because she had lost girl-friends with mastectomies before. I just laugh, 'Oh, mother.' She fell on her way to see me, so she was in a wheelchair when she arrived. So I was really more taking care of her. She couldn't get up and down stairs, she couldn't help me while she was here. My surgeon said that was probably the best thing for me."

Della (47/52): "I guess that other problems come along, and life goes on."

"My family was not disrupted in any way at the news. We had a huge problem at that time. My mother was living with us, my father had died, and she had gone into a deep depression. When I left for the biopsy, my husband had to take care of three chil-dren, plus my mentally ill mother, plus teach school, so we did not have too much time to dwell on my health problems.

"I cried a lot, had many friends constantly bringing in food and feeling sorry for me. Whenever I saw somebody with a sympathetic look on their face, I cried. I liked the attention, appreciated it, but it was hard. The hardest part was coping with my mother during all this time. I was just as active throughout this process, perhaps rested more, but I was a very busy, active person and still am. I wasn't lying around but was keeping house and doing the chores.

"I was probably feeling very low physically at the time, was thinking of my prospect for the future, and wondering if I was going to make it for the first year. My main concern was that I would have no one to raise my children—and concern for my husband, concern for my family, not myself. My major concern was if I was going to survive.

"The thing that has bothered me the most since my surgery is my enlarged arm, which makes it hard to buy clothes. That deformity has been harder to accept than the loss of a breast. The loss of the breast is not visible to other people, but my large arm is a source of a problem to me. There is no lymph node drainage to keep the arm a normal size. Hanging down, the arm gets larger as the day goes on, and every night I sleep with it elevated. I have the hand higher than the elbow and the elbow higher than the shoulder on about three pillows, and I sleep that way every night, which is a chore. And that is for always. If I don't do that, my hand swells up and so does the whole arm. Even at best, it is two inches bigger around the upper arm than my normal arm. It is my understanding that this happens in about 10 percent of the mastectomy surgeries, and it depends upon how much tissue is removed and how much drainage is left in the arm. The arm did not swell until at least six months after the surgery.

"I guess that other problems come along, and life goes on. Other things take precedence in your mind. One thing that has helped me is that I have been called upon many times to visit people who've had the surgery. I know being a nurse helped me, because I had a certain objectivity about it."

Beatrice (54/55): "I hate my bathroom because it has a big mirror."

"Gertrude and I have been friends for years. Her son and my stepson used to room together. We talk things over. I can't talk to my husband, because some of my problems *are* my husband. I hate my bathroom because it has a big mirror, and I see myself every time I get out of the tub. You have to talk about this surgery, and we use each other for sounding boards. It helps. I've only talked to Gertrude, but I feel I am a fairly well-adjusted person, and that is the way I feel.

"I read articles on cancer all the time. Do you ever have questions about nightwear? I hate to see myself flat with no breasts. I didn't have much before, but at least they were there, a couple little bumps. I just can't see myself flat. I always wear my camisole.

"If my husband were to die, I would never seek another mate. I wouldn't want to be rejected. I would be so humiliated. I wonder if age has something to do with it. Now you are quite young; can the young adjust to it better?"

Agnes (48/58): "What can you do once it has been done, but grin and bear it?"

"You're lucky to have a husband to talk to [cries]. After six weeks, I returned to work on a part-time basis. The men I worked for were marvelous. They were so understanding and were really great guys, no problem. They were tickled to death when I could come in with a dress and falsies on. They thought this was just great. I thought it was great too, because it was like joining the land of the living again. I was so tired of wearing pregnancy smocks. A lot of people really thought I was pregnant, so I was glad to put on a dress.

"Sometimes I have five or six spasms a day, and my skin becomes so sore that if I just touch the skin, it hurts. A hot shower does relax me. No, I do not exercise, I am sedentary. What can you do once it has been done, but grin and bear it? You can get a philosophy, but you can sit by yourself with that philosophy. That is what I have been doing, and I don't like sitting by myself.

"I would like to get married again but not just to any old thing. I've been married three times, and I should get a little picky this time [laughs]. Maybe when I'm sixty-five I'll be ready for someone seventy-five. I'll be a good housekeeper. I like men, not by-and-large, but some. To me a man is really the only person I can relate to. The psychiatrist is terribly expensive, and I can't afford him any longer. My son has a terminal illness—not cancer, but a brain thing—and I have a lot of problems with the family, etc. So the psychiatrist at least lets me talk it out."

Esther (44/57): "The worst problem was getting my arm over my head."

"I read more now and understand more. I started to read the newspaper article about you in the restaurant, and my friend told me about it. The worst problem was getting my arm over the head. We put a nail on the front door and I would practice putting a key on and getting it off. It was worse to put on than to take off. We put a clothesline in the bathroom, and I would practice putting clothespins on the line. I would be so tired after exercising that when my husband came home from work, he would have to cook dinner. It took about a month of this. Our sex life was not affected."

Olivia (45/54): "I would love to wear a low-cut dress."

"Mother, father, and my sister were just wonderful, but this is not the only crisis they have gone through with me. I had tuberculosis many years ago. I would love to wear a low-cut dress, and I suppose every woman says the same thing. I wore them before."

Beryl (46/50): "Now in retrospect, it wasn't all that horrible."

"I knew I had cancer and was very depressed about it. I wouldn't have the same freedom to run around nude, I would be ashamed of the way I looked, it would really inhibit me sexually, and all those things bothered me. It had really torn me up. I have never been the same. I have never adjusted to the physical deformity. Now in retrospect, it wasn't all that horrible, but then, it was horrible."

Clara (59/71): "I'm an escapist in many things."

"I didn't cry, but I just couldn't believe it. *Devastated* is a better word, but I am a very highly emotional person anyway, and I didn't accept it as well as you at all. I fought it. I'm an escapist in many things. I'm never free of pain, even now. My arm is quite fat, as they did the Halsted radical. My arm is easily three or four times as large. In almost every dress that I have, I have to put an insert in the sleeve."

Rebecca (64/75): "Now I refuse to listen or look."

"I never read anything about cancer or listen to the TV; I turn it off immediately. I used to listen all the time, but some phrase would scare me, and I did this for six years. Now I refuse to listen or look. Don't be too curious. What you don't know won't hurt you. Don't take it too seriously."

Bertha (64/64): "I nursed four babies, didn't I?"

"When someone told me I had lost a breast, I said, 'So what, I don't need that thing any longer. I nursed four babies, didn't I? At my age, what do I need it for and especially if it was cancerous?' That is how I felt then, and that is exactly how I feel now. But I think I threw out that theory that mother's who breast-feed their babies don't get breast cancer.

"One of the loveliest things that happened to me in the hospital was a young thirty-two year old who was a patient across the hall. I went in to speak to her. Then one day a nurse brought me a red rose and said that the girl had sent it to me. That was one of the loveliest things that has ever happened to me. We have since become very well acquainted, and she and I just had a ball in the hospital. I had different patients in my room, one at a time. One was a very miserable person; nobody else could get along with her.

"I'm just concerned that it should have been found earlier. It must have been there for quite some time for it to have been so involved. The surgeon couldn't have been kinder, and I would never go to anyone else but him. I asked him if I could have a bottle of scotch left at the nurse's desk, as my husband and I like to have a highball. He said, 'Sure, but why leave it at the nurse's desk? Keep it in your room.' He has told that story so often, about that woman drinking a scotch-and-soda after surgery, and he spoke about my attitude.

"I had a very deep depression a couple of weeks ago, as I kept letting it come back to me about not having found this thing sooner, and that still makes me angry. If I dwell on it too long, it makes me depressed. Not the fact that it was cancerous, because that can happen, but why wasn't it discovered before when I gave them every opportunity to do so? Everything was bothering me. My doctor told me I was a good patient, as others sometimes have deep depressions and often.

"The Betty Ford weekend threw me. They talked about her taking a step or two, her bra, and they went on and on and on. I thought, *Boy, I never had treatment like that. I bet they took her right away and didn't make her wait like they did me.* I felt that but did not say it. Also, that weekend was the weekend of our forty-third wedding anniversary. Between Betty Ford and the fact that our daughter didn't call us from Italy, and none of the other kids called us, I just went to pieces and thought nobody but my husband cared. I cried that weekend; I really did. I think that if I hadn't listened to that Betty Ford stuff, I would have been better off.

"I want to get everything done that I have to get done in the days I have. I wanted to take a trip, and my husband has been putting it off. I said, 'Maybe I won't be around next year to take that trip.' It didn't take him long to call a few travel agencies. I want to make the most of every day that we have got."

Daisy (59/62): "I'm just very grateful that I can live a normal life."

"Even though cancer is devastating and the operation is devastating, I'm just very grateful that I can live a normal life. I have no limitations as such, and am able to use my arms normally after the double mastectomy. I play tennis, golf, and swim, so I feel fortunate. I've gotten rid of the 'bad guy' within me.

"I don't think I would ever remarry again. I'm widowed for five months after twelve years of marriage. If I found a person whom I felt would be a good companion for the rest of my days, I would not feel compunction about the mastectomy. The mastectomy would make no difference to me. Now, if it did to the other party, that is something else. Having reached the age I have, I'm not interested in having a family.

"This is why I feel sorry for the young girls who go through a mastectomy, because it is all part of the game—let's say, the sex pattern, nursing a baby. Even when they don't have their breast, we need to encourage young women that now they have their health and still can produce a family; it will be just a little bit different from the normal. The only difference will be that you can't nurse your babies."

Jeannette (43/52): "I am a volunteer for the Reach to Recovery program."

"My doctor had given me only eighteen months to live, so I married my fiancé. Now eight years later, I am a volunteer for the Reach to Recovery Program. I'm helping one woman, age seventy, who is so cute in her golf clothes. I took her a C cup to show her, but she is much smaller so she really laughed. The other woman, age seventy-one, refuses to see me. This has unbalanced her; she's so very nervous and just doesn't accept it. She needs the help of a doctor."

Mabel (41-47/53): "I realize how lucky I am."

"The left arm swells a bit, but I live with it. If I clean or do too much at one time, I get tired. But we must live with it. I can move about, and nobody needs to know that I have no breasts. I realize how lucky I am. I can't find a job, as I didn't work outside my home. I'm not looking too hard. One place in another State said their insurance didn't provide for me, so they didn't hire me."

Jan (32/32): "It makes me feel good that God is using me to help others."

"I still have fibrocystic disease. Rumors are that it can turn into cancer, but I don't know. If I listen to everyone, I would feel panic. I hope to work for Reach to Recovery. It makes me feel good when the women at church come up and say, 'Now that I have seen you, I know I can go through with it.' It makes me feel good that God is using me to help others."

Joyce: (49-51/51): "Live with the inevitable, like death."

"My doctor told me I had two years to live. [I was] very shocked. The doctor said I must have thought something or I wouldn't have asked for a biopsy. I just didn't want to miss work.

"My divorce forced me to go back to school. If I had been married at the time of the mastectomy, it would have been harder than being divorced. Emotion is harder to control than the physical. Live with the inevitable, like death. Cancer is not the worst thing; divorce with the feeling of frustration and guilt made me forget anything else."

Elaine (52/56): "Remember today is the first day of your life."

"My arm is larger than the other, and I can't wear anything tight on that arm. My clothes are all high necked. I was upset but not too much. Everyone in the hospital had been super. My friends sent prayers, flowers, robes, pajamas, candy, and I did not know someone could have so many friends. Someone gave me a plaque that said, REMEMBER, TODAY IS THE FIRST DAY OF YOUR LIFE. Ladies from the church cooked and cleaned my house. The minister just told me everything would be taken care of."

Andrea (39/43): "It is better to be alive, even though not whole."

"I don't feel less of a woman because of the loss of a breast. Between 1961 and 1969, they are what I call my 'middle-escence' years—we laugh about it now; I went through an adolescence that I didn't experience as a youngster with all the pains and turmoil of growing up. A lot of women of our generation have probably experienced the same thing. I've talked to a lot of my friends from school and they have experienced the who-am-I, where-am-I-going thing. I had to deal with this thing, womanliness. I had never been particularly ashamed of my body but not terribly proud of it either. It was just a means-to-an-end type thing.

"I was raised a Catholic, went to Catholic schools under good parish nuns who had talked to me all my life about mutilation of the body, explaining that we can talk ourselves into needing a surgery, and do we really need the surgery? I was also a student nurse in a Catholic hospital. At the age of thirty, which was young, I had my hysterectomy and was having a great deal of conflict within myself as to the need of the surgery, for in my gut, I wasn't real sure. The crux of the whole thing was that we had six children. I had grown up to believe that a woman's main job was to have babies. I could die laughing now but bought it hook, line, and sinker then—that my primary function was to have babies. And then at the age of thirty to lose the ability made me feel somewhat less of a woman.

"The thing that helped me the most to adjust to the mastectomy was the day I woke up to realize that it was better to lose my breast than my life. It was almost a bolt out of the blue. My husband said before surgery that 'I don't care about what may be missing, but I do care about having you here.' It is better to be alive, even though not whole. Plus my husband's assurance.

"In October, I found another lump in my other breast. It did not frighten me like the other one did. They did a mammogram, which was completely negative. I felt that maybe it was just a cystic thing, and the doctor said there was no great rush. So [he said], 'Let's wait and see.' I said, 'Maybe not for you, because it is not your breast, but let's see the surgeon and get the damn thing out.' There was absolutely no argument from the internist.

Again, I had absolutely no fears and feelings that this was a malignancy, but to make sure, I had the biopsy, and it was benign.

"I read all the literature I see about cancer. It is like getting a new car. All of a sudden you see your kind of car everywhere you go. The fact that I have been through it, makes it something to do with me. I saw the article about you in the *Daily Pilot* newspaper, read it, thought it sounded interesting, and forgot about it. Then the next day, one of the girls I work with said she read the most interesting thing about this gal who had a mastectomy and is interviewing women. I told her I read it but did not keep the article. She said, 'Why don't you go see her.' I don't know, why not? So she brought the article, and here I am being interviewed by you."

Brenda (39/40): "The prosthesis is a hassle-and-a-half."

"My daughter says it gives her the shivers a little bit to look at my scar. I've told her to examine herself, but nothing else. I just feel she steers clear of the topic.

"Maybe I've had false confidence, maybe optimism. The doctor keeps telling me, I've got it all; 'You have 80-percent chance of survival.' That is the kind of way I have looked at it. Cancer was discovered early and had not got into the lymph nodes.

"I read the article about you in the newspaper and thought, *That is a good idea, interesting.* Not only stories of other people and what they have been through, but also their reactions to it. I thought the whole idea was great. I hope you talk about the prosthesis as it is a hassle-and-a-half."

Marie (42/42): I've always known I am more than my breasts.

I accepted the loss of my breast from the very first and made no attempt to avoid answering questions when asked.

My greatest adjustments were related to fatigue, radiation treatments, muscle spasms, and regaining the use of my arm. Being a private person, I didn't want people hovering but did appreciate their concern. I did want my mother, trusted friends, and family members around me. The maturity of my husband was reflected in his loving attitude and care of me throughout this ordeal, and this speeded my recovery.

I have loved to read since childhood. Great thoughts by great thinkers have always reminded the human race that God resides within us, and our body is secondary to our soul. Thus, when I lost a breast to cancer, I knew that the essence of who I am still remains. I still know this twenty-five years later.

"I pray thee, O God, that I may be beautiful within."
—Socrates
Greek philosopher (470?–399 B.C.)

"If honor be your clothing, the suit will last a lifetime; but if clothing be your honor, it will soon be worn threadbare."

—WILLIAM ARNOT
Scottish Presbyterian clergyman (1808–1875)

9

IMPLANTS AND PROSTHESIS

*" Earth hath no sorrow that heaven
cannot heal."*

—*Thomas Moore*
Irish Poet (1779–1852)

HAVING ACCEPTED THE LOSS OF OUR BREASTS, we entered the next difficult decision-making stage in our journey: needing to choose between breast implant reconstruction or prosthesis.

We were told that complications can arise in any surgery and that not all women are candidates for implants. Women having metastatic cancer in numerous lymph glands, bones, brain, and lungs, or having other serious medical problems were advised against it. The majority of recurrences occur within twelve to eighteen months after the mastectomy.

Women in a high-risk cancer group were also advised to think twice before having breast reconstruction, because the silicone implant causes a radiopaque shadow that makes it difficult to find small cancers in the breast by mammography. When comparing women, those with implants get more advanced and invasive cancer.[1]

The second choice, offered us in 1974–1975, was to consider wearing a prosthesis, an artificial breast form. This option was the one chosen by the majority of us for several reasons:

(1) some of us were not good candidates because of our health history; (2) we could not afford the surgery, and our insurance companies considered this cosmetic surgery and would not cover the costs; (3) the implant process meant another serious surgery, and we were still weakened physically and emotionally from the mastectomy; (4) such reconstruction was not important enough to us; (5) the thought of damaging our remaining healthy breast by reduction in order to match the implant was too grotesque to contemplate; and (6) we were concerned about the known immediate side effects and the unknown long-term risks.

The Choice of Breast Implant Reconstruction

Surgeon Paul Kuehn offers the following statistics:

> According to a survey conducted by the American Society of Plastic and Reconstructive Surgeons, approximately 34,200 breast reconstructions were done in 1988 in the United States, an increase from an estimated 20,000 in 1981.
> More than one million American women have undergone augmentation mammoplasty since the development of modern silicone-gel-filled prostheses, introduced in the early 1960s. Each year, one hundred thousand women have breast augmentation for reconstruction following mastectomy, or for reconstruction following the atrophy of pregnancy, and to enlarge small breasts. This number is increasing every year. Ten percent of women who have undergone augmentation mammoplasty have already, or can expect to develop, breast cancer. In some area of the country, women at high risk of developing breast cancer have had bilateral subcutaneous mastectomies and reconstruction with the hope of preventing it.
> There is still controversy over whether immediate breast reconstruction should be done following mastectomy. Today, approximately 25 percent of breast reconstructions are done immediately; the remaining 75 percent are done months or even years later.[2]

Not all reconstruction surgery is viewed as successful. Patients the most unhappy with reconstruction are those with poor self-esteem and those with emotional problems unrelated to cancer. These women unrealistically expect their lives to be changed simply by the reconstruction of their breast.

In choosing a reconstruction specialist, we need to seek one who is board-certified, has passed an examination in the specialty, and has special training and extensive experience in plastic surgery and breast reconstruction. We should also check with our insurance company to see whether they pay for reconstruction procedures, which cost between three thousand dollars and fifteen thousand dollars today. This fee is based upon the extent of the surgery: silicone implants versus the new technique of free-flap surgery, which takes wedges of fat from the abdomen, buttocks, or thighs of the woman to use in the reconstruction of the breast.

Dr. Ed Uthman states, "I am against using implants for enlarging small, but otherwise normal breasts." He explains,

> Aesthetically, they look and feel unnatural. Any woman whose significant other wants her to undergo surgical breast enlargement needs to get a new significant other, not new breasts. Medically, there are several local complications of implants, which can be quite deforming and are enough to rule out the procedure for anyone except those who have a severe disfigurement, such as postmastectomy patients.
>
> That said, the current claims that breast implants cause everything from peripheral neuropathy to rheumatological disease have no scientific basis. Although there have been false claims throughout the history of medicine, the ongoing controversy over breast implants is especially destructive, since an unprecedented amount of money has been spent to try to influence the content of scientific literature on this topic.[3]

The controversy and ongoing debate over possible linkage between silicone implants and various diseases continues to alarm women. There is little debate, however, "that implants rupture and lead to deformities, such as rock-hard or misshapen breasts. The argument there is how frequently does this happen."[4] In February 1998, about three thousand women in

Ontario and Quebec won a class-action suit for $15 million against the U.S. company of Baxter Healthcare who makes silicone breast implants. Dow Corning Corporation, the leading maker of silicone implants in the United States, filed bankruptcy, hoping to develop a plan to resolve thousands of claims by women in whom silicone breast implants caused diseases and injuries.

The uncertainty about the safety of breast implants continues. Currently, there are 13,752 web sites on the Internet, covering the subjects of reconstruction and prosthesis.

Our Experiences with Breast Reconstruction

Donna (41/42): "My surgeon is very much against implants, and I agree."

"He doesn't think that any foreign body should be implanted at all, especially after you have had cancer. He does not like it even if you haven't had cancer. He doesn't agree with silicone injections. I knew nothing about prosthesis. A friend brought me a foam-rubber prosthesis from the store. Then the American Cancer Society brought me a soft one and gave me a lot of information in the hospital. I just bought my second Camp silicone prosthesis last week. The salesperson was very nice and made me feel comfortable."

Jennifer (27/27): "I want implants."

"I have a double mastectomy. I want implants for the logistics of holding down a bra. The doctor just thought I was so young to go without breasts for the rest of my life. I like water sports and bikini bathing suits, so I want implants. My husband says it's up to me. He is beautiful. I heard of the prosthesis on the Barbara Walter's program. I haven't bought one yet because I want to see if I am going to have plastic surgery. Now I have been stuffing a little cotton in there before I invest in anything."

Tressa (33/33): "Now I have a choice."

"The doctor told me about implants, and I thought, *How wonderful. Now I have a choice; you have given me a choice when I didn't think I had one.* Since that day, the whole thing has lost a lot of its importance. I do not have to stay as I am, but it is not that important now. I'm still sore and can't wear the prosthesis all day. Some days I totally forget about it, and other days I'm very sore. I need to be totally healed before I could consider going through the ordeal of having implants.

"The American Cancer Society woman told me everything about the prosthesis. She was wonderful. I wear the silicone prosthesis, not a D, as I was never really happy being a D. I'm five feet, one inch, and being a D was the first thing you noticed about me as a person—big breasts. I was never really happy about it except when I would put on a gown and thought, *This is kind of nice at times.* I was always about ten to fifteen pounds heavier, and my breasts, being so large, made me look heavier. I wasn't that unhappy with them and still can wear my D bras, and I don't know why. I kept one that was lacy and I don't know why, but it took me a long time to get rid of my favorite things."

The Choice of Prosthesis

It is very important to wear a breast prosthesis after the mastectomy. Going without or wearing a prosthesis that is lighter or heavier than the remaining breast can cause several problems: (1) spinal curvature; (2) shoulder drop; (3) muscle contraction and stretching discomfort; (4) chest compression on the side of the remaining breast, lungs compressed, possible pressure on the heart if the mastectomy is on the right side; (5) balance problems; and (6) clothing fitting poorly from incorrect posture.

Fitting for a permanent prosthesis can occur when there is no longer swelling and if your surgeon approves. It is very important to find a knowledgeable and experienced fitter. If you are small-breasted, it may only be necessary to use some light padding. If you are heavy-breasted, the weight will have to be evenly balanced so that your bra does not ride up on one side and so you can avoid back and shoulder strain.

Our Experiences with the Prosthesis

Grace (46/57): "I had problems with the prosthesis and still do."

"I want you to bring this out in your book. It stills makes me angry that insurance companies say it is not tax deductible because they consider them cosmetic. They make an allowance for the very first one, but none thereafter. It is not just the money, but the principle of the thing. I think it is the male chauvinistic kind of thing. Our insurance man told me it was cosmetic, and I said, 'OK, I won't wear it.' It really makes me angry. In the beginning, I couldn't afford the Camp prosthesis, so I got a foam-rubber one. I am not very big bosomed, but that one deteriorated. As I got older, the remaining breast sags a little bit, and the prosthesis rides up. Now I use silicone and they deteriorate much sooner than they should."

Sarah (44/44) "The weight of the prosthesis hurts my chest wall."

"I wore a 36B and just stuffed it with Kleenex. I did it when I was thirteen, so there is no reason I couldn't do it when I was forty. I wore what the American Cancer Society gave me at first. The weight of the prosthesis hurts my chest wall. I'm not aware of other things being available except silicone. You need the weight so the bra doesn't ride up."

Bernice (43/44): "I knew nothing about a prosthesis."

"I didn't go to work until I could get a good prosthesis. I just stuffed washcloths in my bra. Each day I did put on my bra because the doctor encouraged me to support the other breast. I had an old bra that was stretched and would fit around my dressings, which fortunately were high enough so the bra didn't bind me too much. That was fine, but I would have to keep adjusting everything because the cotton or washcloths would keep riding up to my collar, since there was no weight to hold it down.

"I knew nothing about a prosthesis before, except what the woman from Reach to Recovery brought. I looked around but felt more comfortable buying from a lady who is also a mastectomy victim, patient, person, so that she could relate a little bit. The first prosthesis was all right, but it was in a little jersey sleeve that fit into your bra, and I found that it slipped around. The silicone prosthesis was worn by the saleslady who was also big busted, and she said it was more comfortable. So I went back in about six months and bought the silicone. I was able to use my own bra both times.

"I first called for an appointment and the saleslady spent more than an hour with me, and she explained a lot of things to me. She was very pleasant, positive, and suggested different things to me, because I was a D cup. She didn't show me the prosthesis for a smaller-breasted person, but dealt with me. I like the silicone."

Denise (56/57): "The salesclerk was more embarrassed."

"I knew nothing about the prosthesis. A lady from the American Cancer Society told me. The salesclerk was more embarrassed than I when I bought a foam-rubber one after two months. I was more embarrassed for the clerk than for myself."

Robin (60/62): "I wore falsies for a while."

"A young teacher was having the same surgery, and I told her that I was looking forward to getting my prosthesis. I never had matched breasts before, and now I could match them. Be prepared when you wake up, your breast may be gone, but when you lay down it is gone anyway and that is the way you will be standing up. I stuffed my bra first with cotton or tissues, but cotton was hot. I wore falsies for a while, the kind you wear in bathing suits."

Vanessa (56/60): "I was small."

"Make sure you're completely healed before buying a prosthesis. When you are small, a regular bra is all you need. They were bringing out this horrible brassiere, which was too big for me with this heavy, heavy thing. I almost fainted when my husband said it cost fifty dollars."

Martha (78/79): "I stuck rags in my brassiere."

"The doctor told me about the prosthesis, but he made me take it back because I got one too soon. He didn't want me to have it until after the cobalt radiation. So I stuck rags in my brassiere. Now I wear silicone and am happy with it."

Ethel (41/47): "I left that rattle in the wastebasket."

"The doctor discussed prosthesis after three weeks of healing. A saleswoman apologized for not having my size because the operation was so popular and she was low in stock. The trip dragged me down, and I took anything. I wear Identical Form. I'm on my second one because they dry up inside. Mine got so that if you shook it, it sounded like a baby's rattle. I left that rattle in the wastebasket. I take a size zero, which is sort of a funny size to replace nothing. I got one through Sears catalogue; it was too heavy and chafing. Then I got one of Kodel from Sears. Finally I got silicone, but that is ridiculous because one size is too small and one is too large, and I'm in between. So I went back to Identical Form."

Margaret (48/49): "The chest wall still hurts."

"I had a difficult time with the prosthesis because it is very hard to match the other breast. The lightest one I found is Truform by Camp. It has been over a year, and my chest wall still hurts, but it is less painful when I have my prosthesis on than when it is off."

Becky (51/51): "She really helped me."

"The American Cancer Society woman came with a silicone prosthesis. She really helped me in that she had a modified mastectomy about five years ago, and only recently had been widowed about one year before. She was forty-five at the time with grown children."

Blanche (47/48): "I didn't know what questions to ask."

"The Reach to Recovery lady came the second day, and I did not know what questions to ask. You don't know what problems you may have as I didn't know anyone who had ever had this operation, had never talked to anybody. I'm bashful. The doctor said she should not have visited that soon. She gave me pads for my bra, and a rubber ball, and pamphlets. The rubber ball is to be used in clenching my fist in order to help me use my arm again. I got a big kick out of the pads with birdseed filling. The nurses were teasing me about how the old crows would follow me around when the sack broke.

"The Reach to Recovery lady should come back before you leave the hospital. The hospital should have a room where you could go in at your leisure and look at the different things that are available, and then you can ask questions. People don't understand how hard it is when you are tired and you go around to different places looking for things. I just ran around, and this was upsetting. I guess it was feeling sorry for myself that these people were not going to help me, that I was having to run from store to store and they didn't seem to care. I didn't get a prosthesis until I went back to work; I just wore cotton in my bra about six weeks. I now wear a Camp. I'm still not happy with the bra. I buy one at one place, they sew in the pocket and it is OK. At another place, they sew in the pocket and it isn't right. I have complained, but it is the only kind they have."

Della (47/52): "Doctors don't know much about prosthesis."

"I didn't know much about the prosthesis prior to surgery. I had a saleswoman who had a mastectomy fit me with one made of foam rubber and weighted with metal ball bearings. This required a special bra. She said she had worn this, and I felt this was a satisfactory arrangement. I went there for three years to the same lady, whom I liked very much, and could also order them over the phone. Then one day she showed me her new one, which she did not buy there, and she highly recommended it. This is made of silicone, which is common now but was not too common then. The best thing is that I could buy any bra. I showed this to my doctor so he could recommend it to other women. He did not know about it either. Doctors do not know much about prosthesis at all, and I say that as a nurse."

Andrea (39/43): "I used Kleenex."

"Prior to surgery, nothing had been said about a prosthesis except that the surgeon said, 'You are aware of the fact that you will need something.' I said, 'Yeah.' Kleenex becomes old hat, as I used to do that when I was young. He mentioned silicone, since his patients had talked to him about them. A very lovely lady in the pharmaceutical department helped me."

Beatrice (54/55): "My skin is very sensitive."

"I had no problem with the prosthesis because I was small chested anyway. After the double mastectomy, my skin is still very sensitive, so I don't like anything touching it. I used camisole tops and sewed in the material that the Reach to Recovery people gave me, until I healed. Then I bought bras already molded. I was filling those with Dacron, and it was too hard. So now I insert nursing pads—[the kind used] when women have babies—and that is all I wear."

Agnes (48/58): "I had a picnic with the prosthesis."

"I was a double-D cup, and when I only had one off, I used Camps and this huge, horrible thing. I used to take it off at night and just sling it across the room it was so heavy. I threw that darn prosthesis against the brick wall and said I hope that darn thing smashes to bits. Then when I had the other breast off, I went to silicone, and they were satisfactory as far as appearance, but they were so hot, and I am warm anyway. I ended up with Extensionette, which were not at all satisfactory because they are not big enough for my rib cage; I am built to be large busted. At least they are comfortable, are not hot, and I just say, 'The heck with it!' I just don't care much anymore. One may be up above, and the other down below. They remind me about it at the office so I just hitch it around a little bit and let it go at that."

Olivia (45/54): "It is easier when both breasts are gone."

"When only one breast is gone you have to match the other one with your bra. With a double mastectomy, I have to wear two different sizes of prosthesis because the side of the simple mastectomy is different than the radical mastectomy side, as far as a cup size. I knew nothing about the prosthesis until the nurse came and plopped down a box and said, would you like to look through these? I was wondering, what am I going to do? The doctor didn't say one word about the prosthesis. The nurses and my friend helped me. I had problems finding a place to be fitted. I wear sili-cone and like Camp because they have the feeling of the breasts."

Brenda (39/40): "I wanted to try on different kinds."

"The American Cancer Society gave me a long list of places where I could buy a prosthesis. I chose a place where I know a couple of gals. I wanted to try on different kinds. I bought an Airway, since Camp Trulife was too heavy, and I could feel that thing all the time."

Beryl (46/50): "Maybe I'm super conscious."

"I had a saleslady who was very sweet and most understand-ing. She has a fantastic ability to make you feel comfortable. I was shocked at the expense. I just got a fantastic one in silicone and it cost eighty-two dollars. Some people don't think it is important how it feels. If you are a single woman, I think it is darn impor-tant what it feels like. You are hugging people and pressing into them. Maybe I am over emphasizing the importance of breasts, but this is me. I've seen several women in the gym without their prosthesis and they just don't seem to have any vanity about it. Maybe I'm super conscious. I've never shown my scar to anyone but my doctor, and I feel embarrassed to show him."

Bertha (64/64): "My first prosthesis cost $42.40."

"The saleswoman told me to wait until after the cobalt treat-ments. She said they had better prosthesis but to wait a year because my other breast may be compensating by getting smaller or larger. I was tickled to put on the one she had recommended, because it gave me the weight I needed for balance. I was quite conscious if my one shoulder was in line with the other. She thought I had a keen incision: 'He sure did a good job.' And that didn't bother me."

Heather (64-65/66): "My shoulders are beginning to sag."

"I was up and feeling better, and there was no reason for my not looking better. Maybe I was sensitive, but the saleslady seemed snippy, so I finally gave up. I was hesitant to tell her what I wanted. I came back to the car in tears because I was so humili-ated. My husband couldn't understand the importance of a bra, so I called my daughter, as I needed female help. I finally went to the dime store to buy foam-rubber falsies, sewed them into a regular bra, and found them more satisfactory. Now I don't have either breast and need two prosthesis. As one side was a radical and the other is a simple mastectomy, there is less of me on the radical side, so I have to put more reinforcement on that side. These are more satisfactory than those that cost eighty-five dollars. My shoulders are beginning to sag."

Julia (39/67): "I've had a lot of problems with the prosthesis."

"I now wear a regular Olga camisole bra or slip. I'm fortunate in having a small breast so I can use the same-size cup for each side. I just wear a padded bra, no prosthesis. My doctor didn't tell me anything about this problem."

Daisy (59/62): "Clothes hurt my scar."

"My doctor seemed to know a great deal about the areas to go for a prosthesis and was very helpful. I had difficulty wearing clothes, as they hurt my scars. He suggested that I wear one of my husband's soft, cotton t-shirts, and that was marvelous—one of the greatest things—and although it clung to my body, I did not hurt from the bra and slip, riding up and down. The saleslady sold me foam-rubber fillers, but I needed a heavy, weighted filler. I went to a wedding and everything was fine: I was standing talking to people and went to sit down. All of a sudden, I could feel all of this filler, up under my chin. I tell you, I got so nervous I nearly jumped out of my skin. I thought, *Oh God, if this is the way it is going to be, I'm going to have a terrible time*, and I was very upset.

"I took them back, and the lady gave me weighted ones—a 36 plus filler. They just work fine, and I wear them now. I work with another woman volunteer who had a mastectomy about seven years ago and who stopped over to show me her filler. She said you lose all sense of modesty when you have a mastectomy, because when you are with someone who had one, you begin to compare notes very easily. She wears a silicone filler, no foam layer like Camp. She said this is the greatest thing ever, wears it next to her skin, and feels just like a breast. I can wear my old, worn bra.

They are coming up with marvelous things. I think the most difficult thing is trying to get fitted with the proper prosthesis."

Jeannette (43/52):

"I use Truform Companion silicone that clings to your body. Other kinds are Airway, OPC, Camp Trulife, Cordelia, and Storekeeper."

Dolores (40s/60s): "Do not use a bra strap on the surgery side."

"I like to be able to help women's assurance because of the time-lapse I've had with no problems with prosthesis, except falsies. I feel too many doctors and the American Cancer Society send women to the specialty shops, which many of us can't afford. I've never known anyone to be comfortable with those jelly or liquid-filled jobs. Just recently a woman was referred to me who had worn one of the thirty-five-dollar ones for a couple years and was concerned with its weight, which was pulling her shoulder down. After looking over mine, she orders Sears's largest—and she has large pendulum breasts—and is so very much more comfortable. Granted, in a tight-fitting, knit dress anyone looking carefully would find the heavy prosthesis better shaped.

"One invention, which all but one person has found most helpful, is not using a strap on the bra on the surgery side. This diminishes greatly the creeping-up problem. Also, a friend who recently tried this said she was able to wear a bra much earlier when her arm was too sore to raise or to bear the weight of a strap. The lightweight falsies do not have a tendency to fall down, in fact, they may still creep up a little."

Marie (42/42): Who ever said bigger is better?

We big-busted women spend a lifetime of seeing beautiful lacy bras, made in lovely colors designed for small-breasted women. Those with big breasts need not apply: please go to another part of the department where we will show you your size—wide straps, perhaps a smattering of lace, neutral colors, and fabric that even a horse would refuse as a harness. Our shoulders bear the marks of these bras, and the mastectomy is just another challenge.

My chest wall is still sensitive twenty-five years after the modified radical mastectomy and cobalt radiation. There is the discomfort of muscle contraction and stretching, problems with prosthesis, balance, and shoulder drop. The sensitive skin sensation is somewhat like having a sunburn, so the silicone prosthesis must be worn within a cotton sleeve next to my body. Otherwise, the silicone sticks when I perspire and is painful to remove. The silicone prosthesis is heavy and becomes hot and uncomfortable. It is difficult for large-breasted women to find the proper size prosthesis to balance the remaining breast. Shopping for bras, prosthesis, and clothing continues to sadden and frustrate me.

Nevertheless, I have never regretted my decision not to have an implant. As with hormone pills, I also questioned in 1974–1975 the possible future risks of such implants. Now, in 1998, we know.

Thus far, I have had to put on and remove my silicone prosthesis at least twice daily for twenty-five years: 9,125 days for a minimum of 18,250 times. But, thank God, I am alive to do it!

> "There is a strength of quiet endurance as significant of courage as the most daring feats of prowess."
> —Henry Theodore Tuckerman
> American author and editor (1813–1871)

"The Lord seeth not as man seeth; for man looketh on the outward appearance, but the Lord looketh on the heart."

—1 SAMUEL 16:7

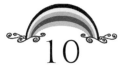

10

DATING

THE MYTHICAL AMAZON WOMEN OF THE 400s B.C. would date men from neighboring tribes for the purpose of propagating their race of warrior women. Sons born would either be killed, enslaved, or sent back to their father's tribes. Legend says that the women would either sear or cut off the right breast of their daughters to make it easier for them to hurl a javelin or send an arrow against the enemy. The name *Amazon* is taken to mean "breastless." Women minus a breast in this culture were honored for their physical strength.

But breastless women in our culture are often viewed with pity, revulsion, and rejection, for female breasts are worshiped as a symbol of femininity, beauty, sex appeal, and motherhood. Many women feel very diminished and unworthy after a mastectomy, which often leads them into casual sexual encounters in an effort to feel wanted. There they often face male rejection. Coupled with self-rejection of their new bodies, these women leave the relationship with wounded hearts and spirits.

Spiritual strength resulting from prayer helps develop a positive self-awareness that goes beyond physical appearance, and it provides the courage to date again within the confines of God's admonition concerning sexual relationships outside of marriage.

Dating will not be easy, but I believe that a woman is capable of a meaningful relationship if she allows herself enough time to adjust to her changed body, and allows her faith in God to define her worth. Her newly developed self-confidence will attract the confidence of worthy men who also want a committed partnership within marriage.

Our Experiences with Dating

Widows

Mabel (41-47/53): "Men I date now just don't call back."

"My husband was never sick until he developed a cancerous tumor in his kidney. That really hit me when they told me after all I had been through. He died eleven months later, and I nursed him for seven months. He was wonderful, but he wouldn't talk to me, which was too bad. I was in a state of shock. He wouldn't let anyone else touch him but me. He went from 220 pounds to 90 pounds.

"We were not newly married at the time of the mastectomies (1962 and 1968), and sex was not the only reason I was married. Men I date now, as soon as I tell them or they seem to know about the mastectomy, they just don't call back. I don't understand that; I'm cured. Maybe they fear recurrence.

"If I knew then what I know now, if I knew my husband was going to die, I would never have had surgery. I prefer death to being left alone. We were married twenty-four years, and he died three years ago today. There is no purpose to my life. Maybe this is a bad day since it is the third anniversary of my husband's death."

Evie (55/56): "Your heart may get broken."

"I was widowed sixteen years ago and was engaged for nine years. My fiancé told me my body was repulsive. I'm still having mental problems. I will never go out with another man. I will not give anyone that chance to say it again. He left me for another woman. I've tried to change my hairdo and go to the health spa.

Your heart may get broken. If it had been with my original husband, he would have said, 'You lost a boob,' and accepted it. I don't think I am repulsive, but it hurt when my fiancé said it. I'm still dealing with that.

Divorced Women

Bernice (43/44): "I probably was a little uneasy at first."

"I have been divorced twice and have had sexual relations since the mastectomy. I probably was a little uneasy at first. So was he, but we got over it the first time. It was easier the second time because the first time I didn't feel that much uneasiness on his part. It seemed to be a natural thing. When I look back, I think he was a little uneasy, but I think the first time you have relations with anybody, you are uneasy. We did not discuss it thoroughly. We have discussed the fact that I was a little nervous, but I felt it was natural to be a little ill-at-ease with any man under those circumstances. He has reaffirmed to me on different occasions that 'Heck, it doesn't mean any difference to me.' If it does make a difference to a man, then I feel the relationship is not worth it. I could have more self-confidence with another man because of this experience."

Sarah (44/44): "It probably would not be easy the first time."

"I have been divorced for thirteen years. Since the mastectomy, I haven't met a fellow yet, but I have given it a great deal of thought. I'm sure sex would happen with a very caring, concerned individual, but it would have to be this kind of a man. It probably would not be easy the first time."

Rebecca (64/75): "Hell, there were no men in my life."

"I've been divorced for sixteen years. The doctor kept trying to bring men into the conversation: 'Go out with a boyfriend to dinner.' Boyfriend! Hell, there were no men in my life. I was single. The scar was ugly. Gosh, I used to hate to take a bath, and I would close my eyes for six months. Even now I think, *Oh God*. I was sixty-four years of age when I lost my breast. Maybe if I were young I would feel different."

Jeannette (43/52): "I married my fiancé."

"The doctor had given me eighteen months to live, so I married my fiancé, and we went to Las Vegas for the honeymoon. We eloped fifteen days after the surgery. I thought, *So what? My breast is not very big anyway, and I only lost a half a pound.* There were times when clothing was difficult. My fiancé was at the hospital all the time with me. This was my second husband. We later divorced because his daughter was turning hippie. My son was the same age and couldn't understand why I was so strict with him and not her, but her father would not allow me to discipline her. We divorced, but his attitude about the mastectomy was that he took it in stride. He laughed and said I was a half pound lighter and still had one."

Joyce (49-51/51): "Most men can't handle it."

"I was married for twenty-three years and have been divorced for five years. I have dated several men, they have said nothing, but most men can't handle it. They are turned off and do not have the same interest. If I'm attracted, I tell them right away just to get their reaction. I don't want to get hurt and personally involved then. Men are interested in the physical you, not the intellectual real person. They want to relate in bed first. Why don't I let him know me first? I can't handle rejection again. I want to be the aggressor and have the upper hand. I still love my husband, but don't want him back. I love him, but there is no respect. He feels guilty because I'm not trained to do much [professionally]. He probably still loves me and is going through a [male] menopause thing, trying to prove his virility with someone else."

Agnes (48/58): "Men have asked, how can I make love to you?"

"I was getting my third divorce. My ex-husband got me to Hawaii twice and wanted to remarry me. He was the only one who was sympathetic, but I knew there was no point in remarriage. He thought it was terrible what happened to me, but it would have been a mistake to go through that nonsense again.

"I think the surgery is the most hideous-looking mess there is. I've run into quite a few little things with men that made me know they feel the same. Granted, these kind of people are not really nice people and there is not too much to them, but who is going to keep on trying to find someone who does care? Men have asked, 'How can I make love to *you?*' If you don't just give in to them, they say, 'Who wants you anyway; you are just full of cancer.' They aren't worthy of anything, but who is going to keep on trying to find someone who is? I need to find a blind man with no arms.

"Oh, I have a terrible temper, and those men didn't leave unscathed, I'll tell you that. I saw them later, but they never knew what I was mad about. I put on a pretty good act. They knew I was angry but not why. They blunder into these things without realizing what they are saying. The mastectomy shocks them, and it frightens them. I think that men, on the whole, are frightened if they are not married to a woman. In the first place, everybody is afraid of cancer and that it might recur. They would be taking a chance with someone who might have it again. You might be ill for a long time and there would be grief. Men tend to run away from grief. We all do, not just men; so why get involved?

"It is a nasty-looking operation, and I think it frightens men. They don't want to face the reality that this happens to people. Then when they face reality and don't expect it, they blurt out things before they stop to think. I told the men I dated that I had a mastectomy, but it still came as a surprise and a shock. I have run away from opportunities that I probably shouldn't have run away from, just because of my experiences. I would do the same thing tomorrow because of the fear of rejection."

Beryl (46/50): "We don't ever discuss it."

"I had a boyfriend and was scared to death that this would make a difference in our relationship. I had been divorced four years and didn't have any commitment from this man, whose wife had died of the same thing—breast cancer—a year before I met him. Now I have cancer and my chances of marriage were affected. I was just devastated. I didn't talk to him about it. He is an attorney, and I just don't have that kind of ability to communicate with him, even to this day. People ask me why, but I don't know why. Maybe one of these days I will, but he went through the death of his first wife from cancer. He didn't marry me until two or three years later when we both assumed everything was OK—that I would survive, there would not be any recurrence, and everything was going to be rosy.

"I would stand with a towel on that side. I just couldn't even stand to walk around the house, even when no one was in the house. It is different when you are married and have a very good relationship with a man. He is going to love you with or without a breast, at least you think, you hope. But when you aren't married, there is a complete overemphasis on physical things. I don't know if you can put yourself in my place, but it turned me off, and I thought it would turn all men off. It was definitely a deterrent. It isn't that I'm highly sexed. I enjoy sex, and I'm trying not to magnify this, but in that area, it really bothered me. It sounds like I'm a sex maniac, but I do have a definite interest, and it has just deteriorated. Now I've come to the conclusion that if I had any brains, I wouldn't have worried about it and just worn a prosthesis all the time. But it took four years to get to that point.

"My sex life has all changed. There is not the freedom to run around nude; I'm hiding in the bathroom, putting on my prosthesis. I leave my bra on during intercourse because I am so bony, and it really throws me off. He doesn't say anything. We don't ever discuss it. I don't know, but I have this feeling that I am doing the right thing. We have been married one year.

"My first husband would have been accepting, but this husband is fifteen years older than I am, and I don't have the same kind of rapport. It is different from being married at nineteen and living with a man for twenty years. Even though my current husband is a professional communicator, we are not communicating very well in our marriage, anyway."

> "We must never undervalue any person.
> The workman loves not to have his work
> despised in his presence. Now God is present
> everywhere, and every person is his work."
> —Francois de Sales
> Patron Saint of Catholic writers (1567–1622)

"Our scriptures tell us that childhood, old age, and death are incidents only, to this perishable body of ours and that man's spirit is eternal and immortal. That being so, why should we fear death? And where there is no fear of death there can be no sorrow over it, either."

—MAHATMA GANDHI
Hindu nationalist leader (1869–1948)

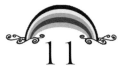

DEATH? FAITH?

"All I have seen teaches me to trust the
Creator for all I have not seen."
—Ralph Waldo Emerson
American essayist and poet (1803–1882)

THE FEAR OF RECURRENCE AND POSSIBLE DEATH after the mastectomy leads to haunting questions: (1) did the doctor get all of the cancer?; (2) did the cancer spread to the lymph nodes and metastasize elsewhere?; (3) what type of treatments must I undergo?; (4) what are treatment side effects?; (5) how much time do I have left to live? We humans have always found it psychologically difficult to accept the reality of our own death, and thus inner peace evades us.

Our society worships youth and denies death. I am reminded of my high-school teacher who told us of the Spanish explorer, Juan Ponce de Leon (1460–1521) and his search for the Fountain of Youth, which he had heard about from Native Americans. This fountain was said to possess magical waters that could restore youth and could be found on an island called Bimini. Ponce de Leon never found the legendary Fountain of Youth; he died in battle when attempting to colonize the Native Americans.

After listening to my teacher, I replied that there was no such thing as a Fountain of Youth and living on earth forever; and who would want to stay young all their lives, anyway? I had seen animals be born and die, and often family members were born at home and died at home. Death was presented to me as a natural part of life, and we were to put our trust in God. I also had wonderful role models of men and women growing old in my family, church, and community. They were not obsessed with youth. The teacher agreed but cautioned that, like Ponce de Leon, many people will continue to look for that legendary Fountain of Youth, hoping to elude and deny the death that humans fear. Our American culture continues to deny death and worship youth.

Our Views of Death and Faith

Many of us were women of faith who accepted death as a natural process, using prayer to cope with the mastectomy and metastasis. None of us wanted to die, and most admitted to being fearful at times. By faith, several of us chose to surrender our will to the will of God.

One woman expressed belief in beauty and living forever, an example of the Ponce de Leon philosophy of seeking the Fountain of Youth.

Those who never mentioned faith, either stated positive goals they wished to attain while alive, or expressed thoughts of suicide, ambivalence toward death, preference of death over loneliness, and constant worry about dying.

Women Who Never Mentioned Faith

Donna (41/42): "I don't know if I could handle a recurrence."

"There's not a day that I don't think about the mastectomy and wonder, *How many days do I have left, how many years?* I'm not trying to be dramatic about it. I don't talk about it around the house. It is too morbid for two people to sit around the house and say let's talk about cancer; it is morbid. I know everybody has to die, but you would like it to be not so painful. I would like to have some grandkids before I die. I don't even have anyone of my four sons, ages sixteen to twenty-two, married yet. I really would not like to miss out on that. You think about these things. For the past year, every day I have thought about my mastectomy but not necessarily about death.

"I don't know if I could handle a recurrence. It took all I had for forty-two years to handle this. It would upset me if cancer recurred in any other part of my body and nothing could be done about it. I think about losing the other breast, but I turn off that thought right away. If I had to have my other breast removed, I think I would kill myself."

Joleen (38/41): "I still fear dying."

"The thought of death is not predominate in my life. In order for a human being to live life satisfactorily, we must believe in two things: first, that we are beautiful; second, that we should live forever. And the mastectomy has a way of destroying these two images. I still fear dying."

Grace (46/57): "I am not quite ready because I have a lot of things I want to do."

"I have had such an extremely full, marvelous life and have had my share. If I died today on my way home, I am still one of the most fortunate people I know. But I am not quite ready to die, because I have a lot of things that I still want to do. I expect to live to a ripe old age for many reasons, because of my own incurable optimism and my own family background with grandparents well over eighty years of age. By the way, I thought you were an MD, not a Ph.D., but it doesn't matter. I'm a skeptic where doctors are concerned, very skeptical. I don't like doctors very much."

Blanche (47/48): "I don't know how I feel about death."

"My doctor told me that my life span is cut down by ten years. I do think about getting cancer again. I think about it all the time. Whenever I read about cancer, it is kind of scary. I wonder if I could cope with it again. It upsets me to think that I will not be around to see my children get married, to see my grandchildren. I don't know how I feel about death. I think I want to enjoy my life as much as I can now."

Jeannette (43/52): "I never thought of death."

"Life has so much for me. I have a lot of things to do, places to see. Look at the positive side. So many look at this so grimly."

Andrea (39/43): "I'm not ready to die."

"I think of recurrence every time I examine my breast, which means possible death. I'm not ready to die [laughing]. I have a lot to do. My closets are clean. [We both laugh.] We have one married daughter, and I want to see my grandchildren. Besides, my husband and I are having too good a time, and I won't want to kick the bucket and see him marry some blond."

Beryl (46/50): "I took a class about death."

"I wasted the first four years worrying about dying. It was constantly on my mind each time I had a recurrence. I felt that this is going to be it, and I am going to go really fast. All I kept thinking about was being scared to death, about being dependent on my husband or somebody to take care of me. I would rather kill myself than go through radiation and deteriorate like I've seen some people. I feared it for a long time. I have sort of adjusted to the fact that I have wasted four years worrying.

"I could have really had a good life these past four years instead of worrying about death. If I had been more knowledgeable. . . I didn't know that cancer doesn't move the way it does in breast cancer. I might have ten years before I will be in a wheelchair, being wheeled in for radiation or chemotherapy. I was just picturing this thing way out of proportion. I don't think that breast cancer moves as fast as people who have other types of cancer, like lung cancer.

"I told my doctor of the time I am wasting, thinking about when and where it is going to metastasize, all these ifs and whats. He reassured me that, obviously, my type of breast cancer was slow moving, or else I would have been gone a long time before.

"I took a class about death, and it really helped me to adjust to the fact that everybody is going to die. I knew this but never verbalized this or brought it to the front. Dying is a natural event, and sooner or later we are all going to face it."

One Woman Spoke of a 'Fourth Dimension'

Clara (59/71): "I look forward to death."

"I look forward to what is going to happen in the fourth dimension. Our world is a three-dimensional world: height, depth, and width. The fourth dimension has no time or space. I look forward to death. We will go into a different dimension, a different type of thinking, have an opportunity to progress. We will go over to that dimension on exactly the same level that we leave here, so it is good to work on your spiritual reaction to living. Believers in the fourth dimension include Emerson, Metterling, A. Conan Doyle, and Dr. J. B. Ryan of Duke University."

One Woman Sought a Personal Relationship with God

Kitty (29/31): "I have tried very hard to get in touch with God."

"As for death, I have wrestled with this for about a year and a half now. I have a lot of different thoughts on it, and it frightens me. I have tried very hard to get in touch with God, and there is something there that I just can't seem to make it. I don't know if it is me, if I'm going at it the wrong way, or I'm trying too hard, or what it is. I just can't seem to grasp hold of real faith that I need to get me through the difficult times.

"I have gone to church most of my life, but have never had the kind of faith I would like to have. I'm seeking a personal relationship with God [in which] when I have a problem, [I am] able to turn it over to God and say, 'Handle it.' I haven't reached that and have talked to my many friends of different faiths, and they say all you have to do is accept, knock on the door, and it will be opened. I'm knocking, but maybe I'm not doing it the right way. I've done a lot of reading. People have brought me a lot to read, and I go to Calvary Church over here."

Women Who Spoke of Faith and Trust in God

Bernice (43/44): "How do we face that many of us aren't going to make it?"

"That is such a personal thing. I've done a lot of thinking about that when I went in for the yearly exam. *What if the doctor finds that the other breast is full of cancer? What am I going to do?* There are times when I think, *Why don't I let it consume me? Why fight it?* Most of my life I have felt this way. I've gotten up in the morning, not wanting to go to work, yet having to go to work, so I'm fighting that. I don't want to be single, but it looks as though nothing is happening there, so I'm fighting there. I want certain things for my daughter, and she is going in another direction, and I'm fighting there. Why?

"It seems that when they took all the cancer out a year and a half ago, they took some anxiety from me that I didn't need, and I was able to say, *Why fight it?* My daughter is going to do what she wants to do. If I have to spend the rest of my life alone, enjoy it.

There are pluses—half as much food, watch anything you want; I'm just jesting. Do a good job, still pick up a paycheck every month. For a while I thought, *Let me go. Maybe there is a peaceful place out there where you don't have to get up every day.* But in my life, I will do the best I can. I'm not afraid of dying. Death is a peaceful place. I won't have to do things that I don't want to do. It would be a surprise to die and find out that I have to do things I don't want to do.

"People have told me that they see me as a happy, carefree person. Yet there are times I have been tied up in knots. I tell myself that I am just getting too old to fight it, so I've decided to sit back, relax, and see what happens. It has been a new world for me during these four years at the end of my marriage. I went *way deep* into a depression.

"If death is the way that God wants it to go, good. I'm a Protestant and am going to church more often now. I started about six months ago. I had a strong feeling about this surgery, that there was something guiding my life and I wasn't in control. That has been the frustration of most of my life—that I have wanted to go my way, and they weren't going my way. I have just about decided that I can't run the whole show. Somebody is going to have to do it. I'm going to have to let go.

"I think there were so many prayers said for me that something good had to come out of it. A lot of things have changed for me and headed me in a different direction. I am really feeling good about life for the first time in forty years. It is God's guidance."

Alice (39/47): "Every day there is a prayer in my heart."

"I live with death and where cancer is going to go next. I get up every day and say a prayer and hope that I get through it. I'm healthy, but every day there is a prayer in my heart. There were days when I got the Bible and read it. I have a friend who helped me spiritually too. I don't know how anyone could survive without having some kind of prayer, really I don't. It is the loneliest feeling in the world when you don't have a mother."

Sarah (44/44): "I took a giant step this morning and went to church."

"I can't remember the last time I went to church. It probably would have happened eventually, but maybe not this soon. I never gave up my religion and always felt that I would live my religion all by myself, but I can't do it alone. I enjoyed church this morning, and I know I will be going back."

Jan (32/32): "Maybe God will give me peace through prayer."

"I fear death. I am a Christian and know I will be with the Lord, but I fear suffering, gasping for breath, the process. I'm dealing with this through prayer. I've been to a psychiatrist twice because of fear of death. My mom was a hypochondriac, so we had illness in the family. Maybe God will give me peace through prayer."

Glenda (55/55): "My destiny is in God's hands."

"Purely and simply, my acceptance is through my own spiritual feelings. I have been very much involved in spiritual seeking for many years. I felt that there was a closeness and help being given from no other word but God. It took me through this, because human beings couldn't, although they were all very wonderful. Everyone couldn't have been nicer, but it comes from inside you, and if it is not there, you are lost and not able to cope.

"I didn't have any adjustment problem, but the only thing that I did notice was I had a few moments, a few days after surgery, of feeling sorry that the whole thing had happened. My poor husband was having business problems; we have had so many terrible things happen in our immediate family, and now this. I thought, *I've got to help him adjust to this and not feel that it is as drastic as it appears.* Spiritually, I knew that it didn't have to be a completely negative thing. People have overcome this.

"Oh, I thought, *This just can't be.* I had always planned to be an old lady, and I have many things to do. Momentarily, I must admit that I just sank down a bit. But then I said, 'If I really believe that my destiny is in God's hands, I must prove it; just live each day.' I now have quite an optimistic view each day."

Tressa (33/33): "God is within me, is a part of me."

"I was not raised in a Christian home. I have formed my own faith along life's way. I see God as life and energy, hope and everything that is good is God. God is within me, is a part of me. I did not feel strongly about any of this before I went through this ordeal. I was reading a lot of metaphysical books, meditation. Those hours in the hospital were not idle. I was totally involved in myself. Some people call it praying. Prayer or meditation or whatever, I wasn't really asking for help but was looking inside myself for the strength I knew was already there. I knew I had that strength; it was a gift to me, and we all have it. That part of us is God.

"There are two places for us to exist mentally for our awareness to exist. One is in our physical body, in the everyday things that we don't think much about. The other is in the spiritual. I had to get into the spiritual side of Tressa and leave the physical alone."

Margaret (48/49): "The fear of death is not there."

"I have what they call 'terror in the night.' Of course, I wonder what is going to happen and how long I have. I have asked doctors how long, and they can't tell you.

"In the past, the surgeon used to be *the* specialist. Then it was the cancer specialist. Now, the oncologists have moved in. My surgeon talked to me for one hour and said, 'Now have I completely confused you?' I said, 'No, you have completely convinced me that you know very little about this disease.'

"He agreed and explained, 'You are exactly right; we don't. I have operated on women with very active metastasis and have known they had to have very active cancer in other parts of her body, and it is now twenty years later and nothing has shown up. Then many women go for five years and nothing happens; then one cell breaks loose, and *wham*. We are stumbling around in ignorance.'

"I am a charismatic Catholic. We had a nine-day novena and asked God for a sign and manifestation in my life. I have felt God so close [to me], you cannot believe it. I always had faith, but it is so much stronger now, which is really beautiful. We had found a tumor, and today it is gone. I can hardly wait for next week for the doctor to see it. It is a miracle.

"Faith has a lot to do with it, and I believe God can make a miracle. I went to Lourdes in Europe. I'm almost grateful that this had happened to have this very close faith-walk with the Lord. I was on the fringes before; I believed, but it wasn't as strong.

"We all have to die someday; we have that coming to all of us. Knowing that someday you are really going home, the fear of death is really erased. I would feel very sad to leave my family, but the fear of death is not there. Maybe that is why I am able to talk so freely about it and am not afraid to ask and am inquisitive now."

Della (47/52): "I am a Christian and believe in life after death."

"I had a close friend who had this surgery six months before I did. She had no metastasis but found she had very little chance of survival beyond a year because of the kind of cancer she had. I went through the experience of death with her and felt very close to her. Because I wasn't having any symptoms, I felt lucky by contrast. She was forty-four and died two years after surgery.

"She was fiercely independent until the very last minute. I was different in this respect; I would let someone help me. But she did not want anybody to help her physically. She didn't want people doing things for her family. She stayed up and active long beyond what most people would have. The day she went to the hospital for the last time, she called a neighbor and didn't even call her husband home from work. This is the kind of person she was. She requested there be no funeral, just a memorial service. She had two children, one of whom is close to me. My friend was also a nurse.

"Age makes a difference. I had experienced many things in my forty-six years and had a full life, a very satisfying life. If I did die, at least I had all these things. I am a Christian and believe in life after death. I don't have a fear of death as I am closely associated with death all the time, being a nurse. My faith was the most helpful, and I have many friends with similar beliefs. These people were the most supportive during the most difficult times. I pray every day, pray for acceptance, for survival while the children need me, but my greatest concern was acceptance: God's will be done. If it is His will that I die, then I hope I will be able to accept it as my friend did."

Rebecca (64/75): "My religion has helped me overcome my fear."

"I did not think of death but did ask the question, Why was I spared? There were three people in the hospital who were younger than I was, who died of cancer, and I was spared. Why? I just felt there is more work for me to do, so I took advantage of the time.

"I retired one year later and decided, *I'm going to find out more about God.* I joined the Episcopal Church. There were things I needed to do: church work, spiritual work, contribution to promoting the field of religion. My religion has helped me overcome my fear. But when I had that biopsy in 1973, I wondered why I didn't handle it better. You can control fear, but you can't help being fearful."

Elaine (52/56): "Be content in whatever state you are in."

"I've never thought of death. I'll be warned by God when I am to die. I have that much faith in him. I have diabetes and could die from that, not cancer. Be content in whatever state you are in. That is in the Bible, to have faith."

Opal (34/56): "I am a spiritualist."

"We believe in the teachings of Jesus Christ, and we believe them literally. We believe the positive things that He said. There isn't any death, just changed forms. Yes, I've thought of death; that would be an honest answer. I felt a little fear before heart surgery, and I said, 'No, the Lord is my shepherd, and he has promised me that I will just change forms. Though this may be the last day of this life's experience as I know it here in this mortal world, I will be in another area, and I will know what is going on, and I won't fear it.' How do you feel [about this]?"

Marie (42/42): I have faith that death will take me home to God.

The faith, love, and joy I felt at being baptized a Christian at the age of twelve has followed me my entire life. I continually call upon that faith to help me handle life's problems. I gather strength from reading the Bible to see how Jesus, in His humanity, handled problems: Jesus cried, Jesus feared, and Jesus got angry, just as we do. Nevertheless, Jesus always turned to God in prayer.

An overwhelming joy and mystery to me is knowing that Jesus loves me so much that He died upon the cross for my sins of disobedience toward God. Being obedient is a deep longing in my heart and a perpetual prayer on my lips, and being human, I often fail. God has never failed me. He saw me through the mastectomy and the double brain aneurysm, and will continue to do what is best for my life. I love being one of the sheep of His flock.

In God's perfect timing, He decided when to create me and will decide when to call me home. It will be yet another journey, and with the exception of deep sadness at the thought of leaving my loved ones temporarily, I will trustingly go with joy in my heart. Many of my beloved friends and family have died, and I look forward to being with them spiritually again. I believe that my loved ones still living on earth will ultimately join all of us for eternity. Jesus has promised this, and God never lies.

I have always loved Hebrews 12:13: "These all died in faith, not having received the promises, but having seen them afar off, and were persuaded of them, and embraced them, and confessed that they were strangers and pilgrims on the earth." I am a stranger and pilgrim on the earth.

> *"You pray in your distress and in your need;*
> *would that you might pray also in the fullness*
> *of your joy and in your days of abundance."*
> —*Kahil Gilbran*
> *Syrian poet and painter (1883–1931)*

"Self-respect cannot be hunted. It cannot be purchased. It is never for sale. It cannot be fabricated out of public relations. It comes to us when we are alone, in quiet moments, in quiet places, when we suddenly realize that, knowing the good, we have done it; knowing the beautiful, we have served it; knowing the truth, we have spoken it."

—ALFRED WHITNEY GRISWOLD
American historian and educator (1906–1963)
President of Yale College (1950–1963)

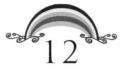

12

RESPECT YOURSELF

"The precept, 'Know yourself,' was not solely intended to obviate the pride of mankind; but likewise that we might understand our own worth."

—Marcus Tullius Cicero
Roman orator and philosopher (106–43 B.C.)

WE NEED TO LOVE OUR BODIES ENOUGH TO TAKE CARE OF THEM, but not allow ourselves to become obsessed by outward appearances. We need to understand who we are as individuals and where our values lie. Each woman must seek the answers to the question, "Who am I?" These answers ultimately reflect our character and inner core.

Am I proud of who I am, or am I ashamed and preoccupied with my body image, which never has conformed to society's impossible standards of beauty? Do I see myself as a worthy individual regardless of the condition of the mortal body in which I live, or do I allow rejection and self-consciousness define and limit the fullness of who I am?

Do I trust my own mind and judgment in making decisions affecting my life and the health of my body, or do I allow others to determine my destiny? Do I succeed by persevering when difficulties arise, or do I fail because of giving up, instead of doing my best to seek and participate in solutions? Does my behavior show that I love and respect myself and expect others to treat me respectfully, or do I permit others to abuse me because I believe that I am only worthy of such abuse?

Do I see myself as a person made in the image of God, or simply as a conforming, unquestioning member of mass society? Am I flexible and willing to face reality, or am I rigid and fearful of change that requires me to make adjustments? Do I value and trust my own opinions, or does uncertainty and anxiety over what others may think make me surrender to their perceptions, out of fear of being rejected? The answers to all of these questions will affect how we feel about ourselves and how we perform.

We must all learn to live with the reality that cancer is only one of the forces that change our body image forever. The other side of the coin is the normal aging process that can be held at bay only for a short time, despite plastic surgery, cosmetics, exercise, and health foods. Our body is aging from the moment of birth and continues to show signs of change throughout our lifetime.

We can either negatively dwell on these changes through tears and fears, or we can positively choose humor, acceptance, and gratitude for what we have remaining: our life, our character, and our God-given talents that we can share with humanity. So where is our faith? What do we value? What are our dreams and expectations? How do we cope with tragedy?

We Women of 1974–1975 Offer You Our Encouragement

We lost our breasts, but we did not lose ourselves. Our experiences have led to the following thoughts, which we hope will help you in facing decisions that arise should cancer enter your life.

Kitty (29/31): "Talk about it. It is no big secret that needs to be hid on the shelf."

"When I told my friends, the whole atmosphere changed. They could ask me how I felt. We laughed together, and now my friends are not afraid to ask how things are going.

"Women need to examine themselves once a month to find it early, but women make too much of their bustline and the sexual attractiveness of it. They should just thank God if they get [the cancer] early enough and it is just in the breast. If a guy has any class at all, if he really cares for you at all, it makes no difference. If it does make a difference, you don't want him. Who needs it? It makes no difference in your sexual life unless the man makes you feel it does.

"My husband has just been marvelous. I really lucked out. I can't see getting all worked up over one breast. That is one of the terrible things in our culture that makes us feel so much less without it. Our mental attitude is responsible for many problems and determines how we handle stress."

Bernice (43/44): "Men should offer support, empathy, and be sympathetic."

"By the same token, men should not be overly protective, because the woman must get back on her feet and continue on with her life. To be overly helpful could do more damage than good. I can foresee a man being completely lost as to what to do with a woman.

"Women should not keep the mastectomy a secret. Be open, because your own acceptance will reflect outward and make others feel more confident. It is not an easy thing, but it should not be the traumatic thing that I think some of the press releases try to make it. This type of thing has been kept a secret for so many years, but now women can accept it more as this surgery does happen to the best of us.

"I became a volunteer for Reach to Recovery because I felt that I didn't know that much about having surgery. I heard all kinds of terrible things. Things I had read in the newspaper, people getting together in coffee klatches. I felt that it wasn't all that terrible, and I wanted to do something to make it, hopefully, easier on other women. I think it is the lack of knowledge, people not knowing what they are talking about, people making things up from the top of their head, assuming things. Now you find someone saying, 'My aunt Millie had one of those, and she died at ninety-three.' We have to make people aware that this happens. People are dying from this, but not as many as in the past. It is very rewarding helping others. Most of the women are very positive, which surprised me. I know they have their depressions. It is nice to talk to someone positive.

"Two young husbands were very open and interested. It is not always fair to say younger men are more interested than older men. It is difficult to include husbands in hospital rooms that are so small when we do our Reach to Recovery demonstrations. It is great to have husbands and even their children attend. Mommy has lost her breast. One child asked Mommy if she was going to grow another. The minute you start keeping secrets, the mastectomy becomes something of which to be ashamed.

"I had a friend who knew she was dying, and she would say, 'Just think, I've had just this much more time with my kids.' She had such a fantastic attitude. This is what I keep running into, and these marvelous attitudes help build me up."

Sarah (44/44): "Women should get back into circulation as soon as they can."

"I don't know of any advice I could give others. What advice can you give to anyone who has to go through with it? I'm better than I was, but not back to normal. I can talk to you because you have been through it. I'm a little nervous today because I have never talked this extensively about this to a stranger before. Women should get back into circulation as soon as they can. Other people should try to be as understanding as possible."

Denise (56/57): "I hope your book gives women more information."

"Maybe they aren't ready for it before surgery, but as soon as they are, they should have help. Maybe too much information before surgery might frighten them. You can tell by talking to me that I knew very little. I want to read your book. If my daughters and granddaughters have breast cancer, I want them to have more information than I had."

Donna (41/42): "Tell her it will get better."

"I don't think I'm the one to give any woman advice, but I did find out by accident that a woman on my street had a mastectomy. I was proud of myself because I had such empathy for her. She is about sixty-five. I wanted to help her. I would never tell her that it terrifies me. I would try to be real cheery and tell her it will get better and she will be able to lead a normal life."

Jennifer (27/27): "Insist upon a biopsy."

"I tell my friends that if they ever have a lump, and the doctor tells them it is insignificant, insist upon a biopsy; they have that right. It is not that big of an operation. My suggestion to women is that if your insurance pays for it, don't be dumb and go home too soon. Stay as long as you can, and get all the rest you can."

Opal (34/56): "Prayer is for our good."

"Women should put themselves in the hands of their doctor and God, and just don't worry about it. In our emotions, fear amounts to prayer. Anything you put a great emotional stress of feeling into is something we can expect to happen. If we want the best to happen, we can put a tremendous amount of positive stress in that feeling that amounts to a prayer. Prayer is for our good. Fear can hurt us."

Glenda (55/55): "If you have a lump you had better do something about it."

"It is not wise to wait to see if something happens. It is better to have a biopsy. It is better to have minor surgery than major surgery. Another thing, the doctor is the first one that has to be aware of the danger of lumps. Anyone who says, "Let's wait and see," is probably not aware of the implications of "wait and see.""

"I have a feeling that this sort of thing brings out the best in people, unless there is someone who is just totally insensitive. People can have a deeper relationship when they have had a crisis. It has served to bring my husband and me closer together."

Tressa (33/33): "Be strong, concerned, and understanding to the woman."

"Suggestions for your book? If I could talk to each one, I would have something different to say to each one. Their circumstances are different. Single, or married twenty-five years, etc. I was single but was borderline. I was engaged, and there would be someone there, possibly. Facing a world that is physically oriented—a woman's body without your breast—would be harder to do alone than if you had someone standing beside you, who already loved you. My advice is to be strong, concerned, and understanding, because the mastectomy victims need it."

Robin (60/62): "Look forward and be a positive thinker."

"I am pleased that now people are letting it out instead of thinking it is a horrible secret. It is not a communicable disease, so talk about it. Some of these people hold it in all their miserable lives. They feel a guilt complex. They don't feel all together. I've heard them say, 'I don't feel like a whole person; I'm missing something.' I say, 'Replace it with something else.' I replaced mine with teaching music, working with other people. I always look forward to the best things. A positive thinker, yes, yes.

"Yes, I have several suggestions for your book. I appreciated it very much when the ladies from the American Cancer Society came in to see me at the hospital. I asked for them. I wanted to see what is to be done and how quickly I could get with it.

"Doctors should not tell patients they are pretty sure it is not cancer; it may be. Doctors should tell patients about prosthesis.

"If I were single, I would tell the men I had a mastectomy, which is what my friend did. She has been newly married for a year now. She had told him, and he was very understanding about it. Some men, she said, weren't. Some of the men acted as though it was a contagious disease. She told men that people who have open-heart surgery had a very bad scar and you don't react to a man playing volleyball on the beach with this scar, mine is only sideways and that is the only difference. I feel that way too.

"We also need therapy groups for women who have had a mastectomy. Metastasis like mine needs to be discussed. It did not frighten me because I had passed the biggest hurdle—the mastectomy. The first time you have cancer is the most frightening moment for you, and you think your world has come to an end there, but no, it has not.

"A book like yours would be a sort of panacea for those who have to go through it. They can read how other women have faced it. It is the future they are worried about. They need to know, as we do, that cancer surgery is not fatal. The book could brighten their lives after the mastectomy.

"The more information the males get, the less rejecting they are. Women need to face it immediately and look in the mirror, because it is not going to be as bad as you think it is. It looks horrible at first, like anything else, but it gets better. Appendix operations leave scars also. The scar is very ugly at first, no matter who has done it. I find that some women are more concerned with the scar than the fact the breast is gone.

"My scar is there, but it is a badge of courage. I don't flaunt it, but if they ask me, I'll tell them. They say it takes courage to go through it, and I suppose it does, but I thought it was a necessary thing to do. I would cross that hurdle, and when the next hurdle came, I would cross that one. Sure, this is my badge of courage [laughing, as she jiggles her prosthesis playfully]. My husband and I always said that if anything like this happened to either one of us, we wouldn't let it bother us. This certainly has not made any difference in our sex. The only thing is that we had to reverse sides, that's all [roaring with laughter].

"Women should buy pretty bras, live the same way they did before. Dress as nicely as you did before. I had to put a falsie in my swimming suit anyway because I'm too small. With some surgeries, you can't wear the bikini-type, but you couldn't wear a bikini-type if you had a hernia operation either. Take exercises right away. I had my arm above my head in about two weeks.

"You mourn over your body while you are recovering. Your grief is there, so OK, good-bye old friend. It hasn't touched your personality unless you let it. You can use it for your benefit like helping others. There is nothing more uplifting, or a good shot in the arm, like helping someone else. Even if it is not cancer, there are a lot of people giving themselves a shot of insulin every day, and I feel a lot sorrier for them than I do for myself.

"You can always look and find somebody worse off than you are. Take a good look at yourself and the scar, then move on. Respect yourself, you haven't lost anything. You think you have, but it is like you lost a finger. It is something you can get along without.

"We have so many sex movies, pornography, and our kids have been educated for sex thrills. Kids have seen it all from the time they are four years old. Remember, breasts are a part of your figure and a part of love, but when they are gone, respect yourself."

Vanessa (56/60) "Your book might help other women."

"They might find a black-and-blue mark on their breasts and not do anything about it. I wished I would have had a book to read. It is like Dr. Spock's book on child rearing. It saved me many calls to the doctor. It was all spelled out for me, and I knew what to expect. If it is a weekend and you can't get to a doctor, your book would help. I am 'anti' hormone pills. I trusted that MD so."

Martha (78/79): "If things have to be done, get it done. Don't worry too much."

Nan (55/59): "Take one day at a time."

"Women need to know what they face afterward. There is a little pain with breast cancer; it does not have to be a lump. There should be therapy, psychologically. I'm not one to give up. You have your low points at times, but I have faith that I will come through. I will take one day at a time."

Ethel (41/47): "See more than one doctor."

"I called you because maybe I can do something for others. Not everybody could answer your call. Tell women to have it done instead of worrying, and to see more than one doctor. My doctor told me not to worry about statistics. He said I was cured after a year. I didn't believe him."

Joleen (38/41): "Become more fully informed."

"I'm reminded that your book shall not be the easiest of undertakings, since it's been my experience that those who haven't been affected directly by breast cancer are essentially disinterested, and those that have reason to be suspicious and therefore are interested, are easily frightened into inactivity.

"But God bless the people we live with and love. Perhaps if men and women alike can become more fully informed about this miserable disease, lives will be saved. It's become quite clear to me that the only device we have at our disposal today to fight cancer is with early detection, and your book could contribute to that factor.

"Newspaper articles make me react in different ways. I was resentful at Shirley Black's article because of her description of waiting weeks after the biopsy. I resent that, because it will influence women in the wrong fashion and the degree of emergency.

They should immediately have surgical procedures as the only safe thing to do. I haven't read in depth about Ford and Rockefeller. Information is good for the general population. It is almost vogue now to have a mastectomy.

"Why am I participating in your book? That is a profound question. I say that the most valuable advice I've heard so far is that if a woman has a mastectomy, she should allow herself to experience and let out all of the emotion that she feels, not to hold it in. Cry if you want. Husbands also need the luxury of showing their emotions, which is even more difficult for a man.

"She should be allowed to mourn as she would for the loss of any loved one, because it is the death of something for her. Recognize it and this will allow for a quick emotional recovery. Husbands need to allow themselves time to adjust and re-adjust. Mastectomy is not going to make a good marriage bad, or a bad marriage good. The whole thing depends upon the present relationship."

Margaret (48/49): "Tell women that most husbands take it beautifully."

"If I had known more about mastectomy, I would not have been satisfied with one doctor's answer. I would never let one doctor make one decision again. Tell this to the women in your book, and tell them to do it right away. Don't put it off an hour; get it as early as possible. I had felt that if I had gone to another doctor, I would hurt my doctor's feelings. This is crazy, but I did. I thought, *Why should I go to other doctors and put myself through all this emotional strain.* But if I had done it, cancer would not have gone as far as it did.

"Tell women that most husbands take it beautifully. A man just does not marry a woman for her breast, and if he is going to feel differently about a woman after her breast is removed, he is not worth having anyway. I met a beautiful, thirty-five year old who had a double mastectomy eight months ago, one month apart. [She said that when] her mother had a single mastectomy, her father left because of this; so it does happen. Imagine the emotional strain that young girl went through, knowing her father left her mother over this surgery. But her own husband has been beautiful about it.

"About 99 percent of husbands are a pillar of strength when it comes to this. For women, it is a devastating thing because you look in the mirror and say, 'Oh, my God, I just can't stand this. Am I going to have to live like this for the rest of my life?' I found the cutest bathing suits and put little ruffles in my dresses, but with all my problems with metastasis, my loss of the breast was pushed into the background. I then realized how minor the loss of a breast is when you are fighting for your life.

"My advice to other women is that if all you are going to lose is your breast, just be thankful that they could do it. Thank God. But when you haven't been there you don't know. Cancer is a lifetime disease."

Grace (46/57): "Women need to make it as easy as possible for family members."

"Everything needs to be done to make women aware that they must act rapidly the minute they find a lump. I have watched three close friends, and in two cases, I'm sure that their fear and their pride kept them from doing anything. They both died.

"Women need to make it as easy as possible for family members. I feel very sorry for families. You can get a lot of good interplay with the family; you can get a joke out of it. Don't misunderstand me, it is nothing to joke about, but there are funny things that happen. For example, my youngest, rattle-brained daughter helped me dress the scar. One day we were marketing and were in a hurry, and I couldn't find my prosthesis. We went to the market which wasn't very full, and we began to push the cart around. She said, 'What do we do if we find your prosthesis here?' and we both laughed. Then I remembered that I had jumped into the shower, put on my bra and forgot to stuff my little deal in.

"I don't agree with Shirley Temple Black about wake-me-up-after-the-biopsy-and-let-me-choose. I would think that one chooses a doctor on the basis of his skill. What is the advantage of waking up and going through the very traumatic thing of knowing it is cancerous? I see no reason for that.

"Be as sure as possible that surgery is necessary. I can't argue with success, because I am alive and perhaps wouldn't have been. I am sure there are some quacks who would be happy to do it for the money. Maybe this message is for doctors, because I don't know how a woman can make sure if the surgery is necessary."

Becky (51/51): "Women sexually secure to begin with will be unchanged."

"On the other hand, women who are insecure in their own sexuality will find this will only be another insecurity for them. I feel very blessed that in my own personal life, I have never been insecure sexually. I have always enjoyed sex. I have always been sought after sexually. Even at my age, I still have men make passes at me, even men who know that I have one breast still make some serious conversations, letting me know they find me attractive and would like to know me better. You know in subtle ways, so I don't feel diminished sexually by the loss of my breast. In fact, I have never felt my power as a woman more, if you want to put it that way. My sexuality and sensuality has never been a problem. The fact that I did have a very attractive figure from the waist up finds us teasing about this at my home.

"My personal philosophy is this: I love life, and as long as my life is able to go on, adjustments for living are quite easy for me to make. My husband lost his job after fifteen years, at the age of fifty-nine. That was a greater emotional shock for him, and he had to make a greater adjustment to living than I did because I lost a little breast tissue.

"If you go to the surgeon and he says you have to have your appendix out, you jump right up on the table and have it out. If he says you have gallbladder trouble and it has to be removed, you just jump right up on the table and don't bat even an eyelash. I really don't know why women take the loss of a breast so terribly. Perhaps it is lack of understanding of their own bodies—a vanity that is focused on their external appearance or an insecurity of their own sexuality. I would have the same confidence in my sexuality if I had to have the second breast removed, absolutely.

"I am participating in your book because I am sure you, yourself, would like to have a balance of experiences, and mine was a good experience and would make a contribution. The most important thing to me is educating women to do breast self-examination and to know what they should expect if they become a victim of this disease. The possibility of them becoming a victim of this disease, unfortunately, is great. If they can be prepared to develop some sort of philosophy previous to that date . . . this was my good fortune.

"I had every single thing going for me: good health, and the right philosophy already developed. I even attributed my positive attitude with the fact that I did not need much medication. I didn't want to be a martyr, believe me, because if the pain had been excruciating I would have said that I needed something. The fact that I could deal with the pain was because I was prepared emotionally.

"I think most men react well. The whole basis for the men's reactions is with the patient. If she feels as though her man is going to reject her, she makes it very difficult for him to help her. The whole burden of responsibility pretty much lies with the patient.

"My friends were also terrific. I had wall-to-wall flowers, notes, and letters, which were unbelievable and I have kept them. They were concerned, but they knew they could depend upon me very well to be resilient and to recover. One of my friends whipped up a lacy, sexy gown for me that tied at the side and was easy to get over my head. The patient's reaction is the keynote. I am a nurse by profession and have been teaching breast self-examination for eight years with the American Cancer Society, and one friend said that dedication to early detection is commendable but this [having a mastectomy] is ridiculous. This was the way my friends supported me.

"A forty-five-year-old woman had a modified mastectomy, and a man she had only dated twice kept calling her and could not find her at home. He called her daughter to find out why and was told about her mastectomy. He was really upset that she had not thought enough of him to tell him. This thing within her—that a man would reject her because of this—was the furthermost thing from this man's mind. They have been married now for five years.

"If you lose a lover—in or out of the bonds of matrimony—this relationship was bound for disaster long before the mastectomy. It is good to find out, because you are better off without such men."

Blanche (47/48): "Face it objectively before you go into depression."

"What has helped me the most is just having everybody treat me as though nothing has changed. I get moods more often and underneath feel sorry for myself, maybe because I don't get special attention at home. Tell women to bring it out into the open and try to discuss it with other people who have had it. Face it objectively before you go into depression."

Della (47/52): "The more you know the easier it is."

"I read a lot about cancer because I am interested in the topic. Anytime I add new knowledge to what I already know, it is helpful to me as a nurse and to me as a person.

"I think what you are doing is wonderful and will fill such a need, because I find that most people I know have not had anyone to go to. I have felt a need for them, as it helps them to know someone who has gone through it. Any information you can get through to people is going to be very helpful. I know being a nurse helped me because I had a certain objectivity about it.

"I work with a nurse—on a shift preceding mine and have known her for ten years—who had so much cancer involvement that she didn't even want to know. She had many lymph nodes involved and went for forty-plus radiation treatments, which is a large number of treatments. She had mastectomy surgery about ten years ago and is fine, with no problems.

"As for marriage, if you have a good relationship and are a stable person psychologically, you can accept this, but perhaps if you had any other problems, this would be a complication. The basic relationship is the key to the whole thing.

"People react to a crisis situation in a certain way. If they were courageous and met things head on, they would meet a mastectomy in a courageous way. If they would be demolished by small things, they would be demolished by this. Or if they were immature, this would be hard to accept. It is a matter of how you cope with life in general."

Andrea (39/43): "Accept the fact that this is better than death."

"Your book needs to tell women about the technical stuff, the importance of breast self-examination, but even more than that, women need encouragement. They need to accept the fact that this is better than death, at least I think it is."

Agnes (48/58): "We must want to educate ourselves."

"I figure that nobody knows what causes cancer, and just because you got rid of it in one place, you can get it in another place. We must want to educate ourselves."

Olivia (45/54): "It is foolish to look back."

"Changes are being made every day, like buying a new car today and tomorrow a new one comes out, and you are sick at heart because you didn't wait until tomorrow. Every time I see an article about breast cancer, I am very anxious to read it because there are a lot of different things taking place; the controversy of the radical, etc. Somebody else is going to benefit from it. And after all, I am better off than maybe somebody else fifty years ago with tuberculosis and cancer.

"That should be in your book: how she can dress so that she feels just fine, and the kind of prosthesis, and where to go to get them.

"Also, women should go as soon as they find a symptom and try not to be afraid because you find out that it is not going to go away. Every doctor should make available reading material to every patient about the breast, maybe even have a prosthesis on hand to show. Doctors need training in how to treat women anyway. I would much rather go to a woman doctor than a man. I have a female doctor for pelvic exams and she is much more gentle than the male doctors I have had. My surgeon just didn't have the compassion for women."

Beryl (46/50): "We shouldn't be dependent upon the doctor to follow through."

"I feel strongly that women aren't informed enough about watching themselves. We shouldn't be dependent upon the doctor to follow through. They don't have the same interest you have, as they have a lot of patients. Women need to know where in the body cancer can strike again, and be watchful of these areas.

"I've attended classes and saw a woman in a wheelchair who also had cancer in the pelvic area, and I wonder, *Is that going to be me?* I wanted to know, but I haven't decided if I'm going to continue the class. She wouldn't accept the fact, felt she was not deteriorating, and was going to beat this thing and get out of that wheelchair. With her, no knowledge was making her survive. With me, knowledge was depressing me. The less she knew, the better off she was. The more I knew, the more depressed I became. So I don't know what is best, to be more knowledgeable and depressed?

[I asked about being more knowledgeable and positive.]

"That is good, too. If my cancer had been capsulated, being unmarried I would have taken the stupid chance of leaving it because of my vanity."

Clara (59/71): "Have more than one surgeon examine the lump."

"I admire very much the attitude you have been able to assume. I'm just thinking of the difference in people. If I had to do it all over again, I would just wish I would have been a better emotionally balanced person. I would just do everything different now. I was pressured by everyone to get it done. I would advise women to have more than one surgeon examine the lump. Take more time. I am the only person I know in my own personal life who had a bad medical treatment. Any doctor who does not want to talk to you should have a nurse in his office that is able to talk to you.

"I feel that I myself would like to write a book of the need for doctors to treat women differently. There is a need for some women to have emotional help. I had seen metastasis from the breast to the skeletal system and had a very good female doctor friend of mine die from metastasis to the spine. I was concerned about the pain, not about dying.

Janice (early forties): "Men should be able to cry and talk to somebody about this."

"I am concerned that there is no program to help husbands like the American Cancer Society has for females."

Heather (64-65/66): "It is better to have two off."

"I was interested, intrigued, and delighted with the review of you in the newspaper, and your attitude. Maybe this could be my contribution: I would like an explanation in your book of some things I still don't know. I would like lymph node involvement explained.

"I know you were shocked when I said I had the second breast removed. You asked why, and I said it was because I had very deep feelings about this and was just as horrified as you at first. I knew you were shocked, because I could tell, even though I know you are going to try to hide your feelings. But I would like the side presented to women that it is *better* to have two off, for symmetry of the body, ease in dressing, ease in swimming."

[I explained to Heather that I was not horrified because her second breast was removed but because she never understood why the second surgery was necessary and submitted without questioning.]

"My shoulders are beginning to sag. An interesting thing happened in the hospital when a small nurse surreptitiously said that doctors don't like us to do this, but after you get out, contact Reach to Recovery. She didn't explain because I don't think she dared to disobey the doctors. Nobody has told me to examine myself, and I feel there is no necessity because I have no breasts."

Judy (51/53): "Talk to somebody."

"I'm here with you now because I had a friend who knew she had a lump for three years and never went to the doctor. When I went in for mine, I told her to go. She went, but died three months later. My daughter was in the hospital, and there was a woman across the hall from her with a mastectomy, walking around with her arm in a sling. I asked my daughter why in a sling, as she will never get her arm moving if she keeps it in a sling. The doctor told her to do that.

"Nobody had told me what it was going to look like, what it would be like, the things you couldn't do, the things you could do; nobody explained anything to me. So I went over to ask the woman if she wanted to see what it looks like after it is healed. She said, 'Oh, would you?' It was just as though she was dying to see something or talk to somebody. I told her maybe her doctor has a reason for keeping her from moving her arm, but ask him. I had my arm above my head before I left the hospital."

Jeannette (43/52): "Look on the positive side."

"Keep doing those exercises. Try not to dwell on it. Feel free to talk about it. Look on the positive side. The young women on the birth-control pill should go routinely for a mammogram, because we really don't know much about the effects of the pill."

Beth (40/51): "Be patient, set goals, and do expect a miracle."

[Beth had died ten days before our interview. Her husband, Kent, shared the following.]

"Beth kept struggling and gave a wonderful fight. Life can be prolonged almost indefinitely today, so women must get this care. Women need to band together and share information of the after effects, etc. This information could be used to help others. For eleven-and-a-half years, Beth had no place to turn but to the surgeon, who was kind and generous. Women need to talk about this. They need the opportunity to talk.

"Beth worked with a bunch of women from Reach to Recovery and would come home and be disturbed about their negative mental attitude. She would say how lousy it was and that they will never pull through, or that if they did, they would be looking through eyeballs that would see a lousy world. Oh, the importance of a positive mental attitude!

"Beth wasn't supposed to live these past-three-and-a-half years. She fought a brilliant delaying action. There is no substitute for a positive attitude, and there is nothing you can do for those that don't have it. She had a sign on her desk that said, EXPECT A MIRACLE, and she did expect a miracle. Our two daughters have been wonderful, real Trojans.

"Beth was on the only diet supplement available, and she knew she was going to die. The day before Beth died, she was planning what she would eat in the restaurant when she came home. Her second project was that she had found a deficiency in the hospital and was working with the hospital staff to correct this. She set

248 -◠- Rainbow of Hope

goals for herself. She tried to stall cancer one more time, that was her attitude. Beth set goals each time of recurrence. One goal was to see our grandson born, then our thirtieth wedding anniversary, then our fiftieth birthday, then our granddaughter, then to take a trip to the Islands. She would set goals that she could see: one day, one week, two months, etc. She missed her last goal and that was to be fifty-two.

"Cancer is something that unfolds; it is just not like lightening striking you. Be patient and expect a miracle. Beth lived eleven-and-a-half years longer than expected."

Marie (42/42): Be aware of the cancer dangers in using the birth-control pill and the estrogen replacement therapy (ERT).

It is fascinating to me that the first injection of estrogen given to an American woman occurred in the same year I was born, 1931. In 1974, it is reported that 70 percent of married American women took the birth-control pill and about 5 million women used ERT. Various studies conducted in 1975, showed an increase of breast cancer among women who had taken the birth-control pill longer than six years. I had been placed on the birth-control pill for ten years because of endometriosis and predicted then that scientists would eventually confirm the connection between estrogen and breast cancer, and they have.

"Think wrongly if you please; but in all cases think for yourself."
—*Gotthold Ephraim Lessing*
German playwright and critic (1729–1781)

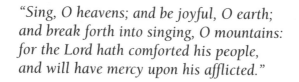

"Sing, O heavens; and be joyful, O earth;
and break forth into singing, O mountains:
for the Lord hath comforted his people,
and will have mercy upon his afflicted."

—Isaiah 49:13

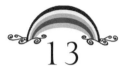

GOD'S RAINBOW OF HOPE

"And God said, . . . I do set my bow in the cloud, and it shall be
a token of a covenant between me and the earth . . . and I will
look upon it, that I may remember the everlasting covenant
between God and every living creature of all flesh that is
upon the earth."

—*Genesis 9:12–16*

AS GOD LOOKED AT THE BOW IN THE CLOUD, I also looked to find understanding in the midst of conquering breast cancer. I gazed at the horizon, saw the red-to-violet arc, and began to name each color after victories I had seen, both in myself and in others along the journey.

1. Through **FAITH** (red arc), we were blessed by a closer relationship with God.
2. Through **COURAGE** (orange arc), I saw a piece of heaven right here on earth, reflected in ourselves and in the courage and emotional support of husbands, families, friends, and caregivers.
3. Through **KNOWLEDGE** (yellow arc) we drew encouragement to continue our battle against cancer. The words of Saint Augustine (354-430 A.D.) helped place suffering in proper perspective: "God had one Son on earth without sin, but never one without suffering."
4. Through **TRUST** (green arc) our faith increased and we chose the attitudes and behaviors that trust instills.

5. Through **LOVE** (blue arc) we stood firm, neither crushed by the present nor fearing our future.
6. Through **GRATITUDE** (indigo arc) we acknowledged God's mercy, seen in the quality and meaning of our lives.
7. Through **PEACE** (violet arc) we gained acceptance by surrendering our wills to the will of God.

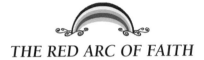

THE RED ARC OF FAITH

"Faith is courage; it is creative while despair is always destructive."
—*David Saville Muzzey*
American historian and educator (1870–1965)

I entered my stormy battle against breast cancer by putting on the full armour of God, as described by the apostle Paul:

> Wherefore take unto you the whole armour of God, that ye may be able to withstand in the evil day, and having done all, to stand. Stand therefore, having your loins girt about with truth, and having on the breastplate of righteousness; And your feet shod with the preparation of the gospel of peace; Above all, taking the shield of faith, wherewith ye shall be able to quench all the fiery darts of the wicked. And take the helmet of salvation, and the sword of the Spirit, which is the word of God; Praying always with all prayer and supplication to the Spirit, and watching thereunto with all perseverance. (Eph. 6:13–18).

Although I have wondered why my life was spared after the mastectomy in 1974 and again in 1995 after the double brain aneurysm, I know that my life and death are in God's hands. He has a purpose for my life and I do not need to understand the why of it.

A contemporary of ours, Helen Keller (1880–1968), endured blindness and deafness, yet said, "My blindness is part of the working out of God's divine plan. My incompleteness he transmutes into a gift of hope to others." I also believe that God will use my incompleteness, resulting from the mastectomy, as a gift of hope and encouragement to others.

With absolute trust in God, I do not fear death, for Christ conquered death on the cross for my sins: "Death is swallowed up in victory. O death, where is thy sting? O grave, where is thy victory?" (1 Cor. 15:54–55). For me, as with rainbows, this is a beautiful and joyful awareness of God's love for us.

I found the red arc of faith and was blessed by a closer relationship with God. By surrendering my will to the will of God, I was rewarded with perseverance, optimism, strength, comfort, and courage.

THE ORANGE ARC OF COURAGE

"The bravest thing you can do when you are not brave is to profess courage and act accordingly."

—*Corra May White Harris*
American author (1869–1935)

The moment we are brave enough to face and accept the reality of our own inevitable death sometime in the future, we are then set free to live a meaningful life in the present.

Courage is almost as individualized as fingerprints, for no two people react to danger in the exact same manner or with the exact same intensity. Often, we can be inspired by others, but the decision to act courageously is a solo choice at any given time.

We seventy women chose to share our intimate and honest feelings concerning personal experiences with breast cancer and its aftermath. We were willing to relive the pain of remembrance and tell our stories, because we hoped to help other women who may face breast cancer and its consequences. You will be the judge of individual courage. Many of us saw courage around us in our children, husbands, families, friends, and medical caregivers.

Children returned their parent's love, such as Tina (30) who saw her mother, Becky (51/51) as a "fantastic person" of courage: "If it happens to me, I hope I can be as strong as my mother."

Some of us had *courageous husbands* who lovingly encouraged us each step along our journey. They did their best to assure us that they understood our grief, but they also wanted us to understand that they were more concerned about losing us than about losing a breast. Such husbands were described as "marvelous, accepting, sensitive, tender, calming, kind, wonderful, sharing, and honest in their feelings." Glenda (55/55) speaks for us when she said, "The very best has come out of him." These husbands inspired their wives toward courage because of their own personal inner strength.

Families and friends showered us with love in a variety of ways. They prayed for us, cleaned our homes, cooked our food, cared for our children, sent cards and gifts of encouragement, visited our hospital bedsides, used humor to uplift our spirits, and supported us when we returned to our jobs. They bravely embraced our bodies and our pain. I viewed my loving family and friends as a piece of heaven right here on earth.

Caregivers in the medical profession who helped many of us the most were those whose own bravery kept them knowledgeable, well-trained, up-to-date, competent, and patient. They answered our questions and had a bedside manner. We saw genuine compassion on their faces, felt it in their touch, and heard it in their voices.

God worked through our caregivers to sustain us. These doctors, surgeons, nurses, oncologists, anesthesiologists, technicians, hospital staffs, and researchers continued on their courageous journey, hoping to help save other lives. My prayer for them remains that "The Lord watch between me and thee, when we are absent one from another" (Gen. 31:49).

I bonded with those who courageously sustained me, and they continue to be with me in the orange arc of courage.

THE YELLOW ARC OF KNOWLEDGE

"I keep six honest serving-men. (They taught me all I knew): Their names are What and Why and When and How and Where and Who."
—Rudyard Kipling
English author (1865–1936)

How informed were we seventy women about breast cancer in 1974–1975? What did we want to know? When did we want to know it? The amount of knowledge sought or refused depended upon the viewpoint of each woman. This is true of women today.

- Becky (51/51) represents women who already knew a great deal about the mastectomy because of their affiliation with the medical profession, either as nurses, or as wives and relatives of doctors.
- Daisy (59/62) represents women whose well-informed doctors thoroughly explained the mastectomy choices and treatments.
- Grace (46/57) represents women whose doctors did not discuss surgery alternatives, and who did not ask questions of their doctors.
- Alice (39/47) represents women too fearful to ask questions.
- Nan (55/59) represents women who did not know what questions to ask.
- Margaret (48/49) represents women who asked their doctors to withhold information because they wanted to remain hopeful going into surgery.
- Bernice (43/44) represents women who did not feel the need for much information because of their faith in their doctor's knowledge.
- Joleen (38/41) represents women who left decisions concerning the mastectomy entirely to doctors they trusted.
- Fay (?) represents women who chose death over any treatment.
- I represent women who knew very little about the mastectomy but who immediately sought information about choices before agreeing to surgery and treatment. We wanted to be a part of the decision-making process that so profoundly affected our lives.

It is now twenty-five years later, and I continue to fervently believe that every woman must take an active role in gaining the information she will need to help save her own life. Knowledge is power and Rudyard Kipling's "six honest serving-men" are needed allies that will teach us about cancer. We must tenaciously ask what? why? when? how? where? and who? For cancer is a lifetime disease with no known cure thus far.

Answered questions lead to early detection. Until a cure for cancer is finally found, women today must have inquiring minds, asking many of the same questions we asked in 1974–1975, particularly with the constraints under current HMOs trying to balance cost-containment versus quality care of the patient.

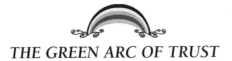

THE GREEN ARC OF TRUST

"Trust God where you cannot trace Him. Do not try to penetrate the cloud He brings over you; rather look to the bow that is in it. The mystery is God's; the promise is yours."

—*John Ross Macduff*
Scottish Presbyterian clergyman (1818–1895)

I learned that the best way for me to handle my fear upon hearing the words *breast cancer* was to attack cancer head-on by asking questions that led to honest reflection. What is important to me? What do I fear? How can I free myself of my anxieties? What actions must I take? Who do I trust to help me? I was among those women who used such introspection and drew strength from a deeper understanding of self.

Many of us trusted our families, our doctors and caregivers, and our friends. I and others had an abiding faith in God, and we confidently placed our lives and our deaths in His hands. With trust in our hearts, we turned to God in prayer and drew comfort from reading our Bibles. "Trust in the Lord with all thine heart; and lean not unto thine own understanding. In all ways acknowledge him and he shall direct thy paths" (Prov. 3:5–6).

I could not alter the circumstance of having breast cancer, but I could, with the help of God, alter my attitudes and behaviors. My faith increased as I claimed as my own a prayer that King David of the Old Testament offered to God:

> Cause me to hear thy lovingkindness in the morning; for in thee do I trust: cause me to know the way wherein I should walk; for I lift up my soul unto thee. . . . For I am thy servant. (Ps. 143:8, 12).

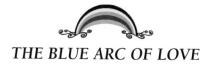

THE BLUE ARC OF LOVE

"The heart of him who truly loves is a paradise on earth; he has God in himself, for God is love."

—*Felicite Robert de Lamennais*
French priest and philosopher (1782–1854)

Love enabled most of us to value ourselves more than we valued our breasts, and we chose a life after our mastectomies that reflected the philosophy of Robin (60/62): "Look forward and be a positive thinker. My scar is a badge of courage. I say replace your loss with something else, such as helping others."

Some could not go beyond a worldly definition of love, and defined themselves by their breasts. When the mastectomy entered the lives of these women, a healthy perspective of the value of life was lost, and the part became more important than the whole. Because they were unable to love and value themselves, their despair led to failed relationships.

Loving myself enabled me to refuse to be at war with who I became physically. I refused to be preoccupied and dissatisfied with my appearance, refused to hide from reality, refused to allow the fashion of the day to determine my worth, and refused to be limited by the secular world's approval of who is worthy of love.

Knowing myself to be loved by God, I felt secure with His promise of unconditional eternal love: "He hath said, I will never leave thee, nor forsake thee" (Heb. 13:5).

I chose to hold onto hope and was not willing to give up in my fight against cancer. I chose to befriend and love myself and my changed body. I was then prepared to follow the inspiration given by the Roman emperor and philosopher Marcus Aurelius (121–180 A.D.), of standing firm against any misfortune:

> Be like the cliff against which the waves continually break; but it stands firm and tames the fury of the water around it. . . . I am neither crushed by the present nor fearing the future. . . . Remember, too, this maxim on every occasion that tempts you to vexation: This is not a misfortune; and to bear it nobly is good fortune.[1]

THE INDIGO ARC OF GRATITUDE

"God has two dwellings: one in heaven, and the other in a meek and thankful heart."

—*Izaak Walton*
English biographer and author (1593–1683)

I awoke from surgery with a feeling of gratitude at being alive! As my recuperation began, hope propelled me toward an optimistic future full of new possibilities. I was grateful for God's mercy, grateful to those who worked to keep me alive, and grateful to those who wept when I wept and rejoiced when I rejoiced. My will to live and my zest for life were the winning combination that helped me focus on recovery. I did not look back. I did not give up, I did not lose heart, because faith in God was my constant companion.

Although we women had suffered and did not know how much more time would be allotted us by God, many of us gratefully acknowledged that life was worth fighting for, and continued our battle against cancer.

It is not the length of my life but the quality and meaning of my experiences that are important. Did the reflections of my life enrich, uplift, and encourage others as we journey together on earth? If the answer to this question is yes, then this is a grateful life worth living, worth fighting to keep.

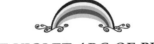

THE VIOLET ARC OF PEACE

"Peace I leave with you, my peace I give unto you: not as the world giveth, give I unto you. Let not your heart be troubled, neither let it be afraid."

—*John 14:27*

Peace of mind is as multifaceted as a rainbow and as complex as the people who seek serenity of spirit. Even though a seven-color rainbow may be visible after a storm, science tells us there also exists an entire spectrum of colors—beyond the red-to-violet arc—that is invisible to the naked eye. Just because we are unable to see these additional colors, does not mean they are not there.

In the turbulent storm that followed our journey with breast cancer, the pot of gold we sought at the end of the rainbow was to be free from cancer, and to have the peace of mind that often eluded us.

Where and how do we find such peace of mind? Over three hundred years ago, the French author and moralist, Duc Francois de la Rochefoucauld (1613–1680) announced, "When we do not find peace within ourselves, it is vain to seek it elsewhere."

Around the turn of the seventeenth century, the English clergyman Matthew Henry (1661–1714) stood firm: "Peace is such a precious jewel that I would give anything for it but the truth."

Over two hundred years later, the Hindu nationalist leader, Mahatma Gandhi (1869–1948) agreed: "The way of peace is the way of truth. Truthfulness is even more important than peacefulness. Each one has to find his peace from within. And peace, to be real, must be unaffected by outside circumstances."

Mother Teresa had no doubt of the way to inner peace: "What makes the difference is total surrender to God. To accept whatever He gives, and to give whatever it takes with a big smile. This is the surrender to God."

My inner peace comes in knowing I am so loved by God that He will never desert me, no matter the circumstances. The experiences of my life have shown me the truth of this reality. I cannot escape the love of God. Over one hundred years ago, poet Francis Thompson (1859–1907) wrote his legendary poem, "The Hound of Heaven", which tells me that no matter how I may try to hide from God, I am never successful, because God continues to search for me.

In order to live at peace with myself, I had to assume the attitude of self-acceptance and self-respect for the person I was before the mastectomy, and the person I became afterward. I faced what had to be done to save my life and left the results in the hands of God. This took a deliberate act of will.

Attaining serenity was not a once-and-for-all-time accomplishment. Indeed, daily I faced my demons of fear, while I lifted my prayers to God for the strength and courage to face the truth of my prognosis and radiation treatments. The "Serenity Prayer" of St. Francis became another act of will and remains so to this day: "O Lord, grant me the strength to change the things that need changing, the courage to accept the things that cannot be changed, and the wisdom to know the difference."

There could be no sustaining inward calm for me unless I was able to make peace with death. Where did the strength come from to accept my mortality and to endure tragedy? From within me. How did I acquire the ability to accept God's will for my life? By surrendering my life to God, through faith that leads to prayer and a trusting personal relationship with God. Many who believe in God understand this surrender.

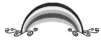

THE END OF MY RAINBOW JOURNEY WITH SEVENTY WOMEN

"Not in the achievement, but in the endurance of the human soul, does it show its divine grandeur, and its alliance with the infinite God."
—Edwin Hubbel Chapin
American clergyman (1814–1880)

From the midst of our suffering, we volunteered to come together in 1974–1975, sharing our breast-cancer experiences, with the desire to develop a book that would provide hope and encouragement for others. We had the commonality of a mastectomy but brought different experiences, as we came from different backgrounds.

We were nurses, teachers, artists, college students, business executives, entrepreneurs, homemakers, saleswomen, waitresses, secretaries, typists, clerks, socialites, a professional cook, a laundry worker, and a cerebral palsy victim. Our ranks included married, divorced, widowed, and single women between the ages of twenty-seven and seventy-nine.

No one can judge the sufferings of another person. We learned what we could endure as individuals and sometimes were surprised by our own responses to the mastectomy. During the interviews, each woman was in her own stage of grieving the death of her breast(s): denial, anger, bargaining, depression, and acceptance—the five stages defined by Dr. Elisabeth Kubler-Ross in her books on death and dying.

> "Patients who are in the stage of acceptance show a very outstanding feeling of equanimity and peace. There is something dignified about these patients, while the people in the stage of resignation [depression and anger] are very often indignant, full of bitterness and anguish, and very often express the statement, 'What's the use? I'm tired of fighting.' It's a feeling of futility, of uselessness and lack of peace, which is quite easily distinguishable from a genuine stage of acceptance."[2]

The grieving stage of resignation [depression and anger]

The women I interviewed who were in the stages of denial and of resignation expressed their bitterness in a variety of ways:

- Refusing to look at themselves in the mirror
- Threatening to break every mirror in the house
- Showing hatred for their body by hiding behind a towel
- Closing their eyes while dressing and refusing to look at their scar
- Shouting and crying hysterically
- Fits of swearing
- Refusing to open the door to neighbors
- Telling their husbands to leave them and find a young woman with two breasts
- Refusing to have sex in the light or take showers with husbands anymore
- Hating not being able to wear low-cut clothing and show their breasts
- Wanting to die
- Threatening suicide.

I personally did not experience such forms of denial, depression, and anger at the loss of my breast. Contrary to shunning my body, I deliberately looked at myself nude in the bathroom mirror daily in order to become accepting of my changed form, and to prepare myself to show my husband the scar shortly after surgery. At no time was I in the state of denial. Accepting reality, and permitting myself to cry and grieve, helped hasten my full recovery.

Because I believed it was my responsibility to set a positive tone of acceptance for the mastectomy and for the rest of my life, I worked toward this goal, and found myself to be in the stage of acceptance before beginning the interviews six weeks after my surgery. Although not relating to the expressions and behavior of denial during these interviews, I experienced sorrow and compassion for those bearing the pain of such thoughts.

The stage of acceptance [equanimity and peace]

When interviewed, women in this stage discussed positive attitudes, situations, and personal growth which showed their acceptance of the mastectomy:

- I came to know and like myself better.
- I will never take this day for granted.
- I dwell on positive thoughts, just feeling life.
- I'm not one to give up.
- I have surrendered control of my life to God.
- I'm a fighter, not less feminine.
- I remain hopeful with a strong faith.
- I believe in a miracle.
- I'm grateful to live a normal life.
- I realize how lucky I am.
- I'm now a stronger person.
- My scar is beautiful.
- I enjoy helping others: Reach to Recovery, and church activities.
- I can smile and make jokes about it: both prosthesis fell on the ground when gardening; organist forgot her prosthesis and was fined by her friends; daughter teased her mother that they might find her prosthesis in the grocery store when her mom forgot to wear it.

I also experienced leaving home without the prosthesis. Luckily, I was driving alone on my way to teach and just happened to spill some tea on my blouse. Reaching down to brush away any spots, I found my silicone friend missing and laughed. It is wonderfully liberating to be able to laugh at such preposterous situations, and several of us knew this.

We also knew that every day was ever so precious. Along our journey, five of the seventy women died in 1975, shortly after being interviewed, as cancer had metastasized throughout their bodies: Kitty (29/31), Janice (early forties), Margaret (48/49), Beth (40/51), and Nan (55/59). In 1993, at the age of eighty-five, Julia (39/67) died from complications of hip surgery unrelated to cancer, and had survived her modified radical mastectomy for forty-six years. All six embarked on yet another journey—the one home to God.

They died as women of faith and could say, as did apostle Paul: "I have fought a good fight, I have finished my course, I have kept the faith" (2 Tim. 4:7).

How many of the remaining sixty-four women have survived these past twenty-five years is unknown to me. Our youngest, Jennifer (27/27), would now be fifty-two. Our most senior, Martha (78/79), would now be 104 years of age, which is possible but unlikely. Whether living or dead, these women are very dear to my heart and have left us words of encouragement and insight as represented below:

- "See more than one doctor." Ethel (41/47)
- "Have more than one surgeon examine the lump." Beryl (46/50)
- "Become more fully informed." Joleen (38/41)
- "The more you know the easier it is." Della (47/52)
- "We must want to educate ourselves." Agnes (48/58)
- "Your book might help other women." Vanessa (56/60)
- "We shouldn't be dependent upon the doctor to follow through." Beryl (46/50)
- "If you have a lump you had better do something about it." Glenda (55/55)
- "Insist upon a biopsy." Jennifer (27/27)
- "If things have to be done, get them done. Don't worry." Martha (78/79)

- "Face it objectively before you go into depression."
  Blanche (47/48)
- "Accept the fact that this is better than death."
  Andrea (39/43)
- "Take one day at a time." Nan (55/59)
- "Prayer is for our good." Opal (34/56)
- "It is foolish to look back." Olivia (45/54)
- "Look forward and be a positive thinker." Robin (60/62)
- "Look on the positive side." Jeannette (43/52)
- "It will get better; you will be able to lead a normal life."
  Donna (42/42)
- "Talk about it. It is no big secret that needs to be hid on
  the shelf." Kitty (29/31)
- "Be open, because your own acceptance will reflect outward and make others feel more confident."
  Bernice (43/44)
- "Women need to make it as easy as possible for family
  members." Grace (46/47)
- "Be strong, concerned, and understanding of the women."
  Tressa (33/33)
- "Tell women that most husbands take it beautifully."
  Margaret (48/49)
- "Women sexually secure to begin with will be
  unchanged." Becky (51/51)
- "Men should be able to cry and talk to somebody about
  this." Beryl (46/50)
- "Be patient, set goals, and do expect a miracle."
  Beth (40/51)
- "Be aware of the cancer dangers in using the birth-control
  pill and estrogen replacement therapy."
  Marie (42/42)

I saw these remarkable women doing the best they could at this juncture in their lives.

My prayer for each was that God would bless us with the personal peace and acceptance like that reflected in the life of the apostle Paul, a man of God I particularly esteem:

Be careful [worried] for nothing; but in every thing by prayer and supplication with thanksgiving let your requests be known unto God. And the peace of God, which passeth all understanding, shall keep your hearts and minds through Christ Jesus. Finally, brethren, whatsoever things are just, whatsoever things are pure, whatsoever things are lovely, whatsoever things are of good report; if there be any virtue, and if there be any praise, think on these things. . . . for I have learned, in whatsoever state I am, therewith to be content. I know both how to be abased, and I know how to abound: every where and in all things I am instructed both to be full and to be hungry, both to abound and to suffer need. I can do all things through Christ which strengtheneth me. (Phil. 4:6-13).

Our yesterdays do follow us into tomorrow. I honor and lovingly remember these brave women. I have faithfully presented their thoughts in our book. We shared a divine grandeur, for we fought breast cancer in the best way we knew at the time, and we tasted victory. This is the essence of life. Not all was sadness. Much was joy.

> *"The joys I have possessed are ever mine;*
> *out of thy reach, behind eternity,*
> *hid in the sacred treasure of the past,*
> *but blest remembrance brings them hourly back"*
> *—John Dryden*
> *English poet (1631–1700)*

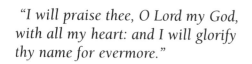

*"I will praise thee, O Lord my God,
with all my heart: and I will glorify
thy name for evermore."*

—P<small>SALM</small> 86:12

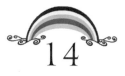

TWENTY-FIVE YEARS
OF SURVIVAL

"We live in deeds, not years; in thoughts, not breaths; in feelings, not in figures on the dial; we should count time by heart-throbs. He most lives who thinks most, feels the noblest, acts the best."

—*Gamaliel Bailey*
American Editor and abolitionist (1807–1859)

THE WOMEN INTERVIEWED TWENTY-FIVE YEARS AGO were asked, "What helped you the most to accept/adjust to cancer and the mastectomy?" I posed no questions to them concerning God, but numerous women gave Him the credit for seeing them through, and I am such a woman.

In 1974, two important challenging events affected my life: on February 11, receiving my Doctor of Philosophy Degree in Education from Claremont Graduate University in California; and on September 24, experiencing breast cancer, resulting in a modified radical mastectomy. Both events are examples of life's achievements and unpredictability. I found commonality in what was needed for me to meet both challenges:

- The personal optimism that said, *I can do this.*
- The commitment to persevere when situations became stressful.
- The determination to reach a positive goal despite road-blocks.

- The faith that God would accompany, protect, and strengthen me.
- The support of my loving husband, who always encouraged me to do my best.
- The ability to laugh at myself in the midst of failures and successes.
- The courage to forgive myself and others.
- The joy of small victories earned step by step.

These characteristics made it possible for me, at the age of twenty-nine, to begin working my way through college to achieve the doctorate, and later, at the age of forty-two, to face and survive the reality of breast cancer.

Some women feel destroyed after a mastectomy, unable to feel hope, but I have never lost sight of hope and have lived a normal, productive life these past twenty-five years, a life filled with opportunities for joy and contribution. More and more women are surviving breast cancer today and experiencing wonderful achievements.

The things that were of value to me in my youth still define me today: the rewards of loving, sharing, and helping others; the love of learning; the joy of trying to live in a manner that honors God; and the blessings of God's merciful forgiveness for the many times I have failed Him. This is a life worth living, whatever its duration.

The loss of a breast did not end my world, but it did remind me of the brevity of life. So I stepped out again in faith and went about my daily living. I never asked, "Why me?", and took every day as a gift from God, trying to use that gift to enrich the lives of others. I felt a special, kindred spirit with Beth (40/51), who continued to set numerous goals for herself, and kept a sign on her desk that said, EXPECT A MIRACLE. Our philosophy of life was the same.

I credit my faith, my positive attitude, and my beloved husband, Bill, for helping me recover from breast cancer. I was shortly afterward able to return to my position as a certificated personnel assistant in the Huntington Beach Union High School District, working half days, while taking radiation treatments. I then assumed duties as assistant director of their adult school, later resigning in order to achieve another goal—that of purchasing real estate and, in 1978, starting an antique-and-gift business called Moods and Memories. Five years later, in 1983, another goal was achieved when Bill retired as marketing manager for Hughes Aircraft and started his own business, Solid State Sales, as a sales representative for semiconductor manufacturers.

Yes, there is hope after mastectomy! Yes, there are many opportunities for accomplishment if we each look for our own rainbow of hope. I did not dwell on thoughts of death, but threw myself into the act of living, with a hunger in my heart to honor God.

Breast cancer did not stop me from the excitement of learning and discovery, nor did Bill and I allow the mastectomy to interfere with our goals of business trips and worldwide travel with family members, including three cruises to places such as Finland, Sweden, Norway, Denmark, Russia, Japan, Hong Kong, Thailand, Singapore, Taiwan, England, Australia, New Zealand, Scotland, Alaska, Italy, Greece, Turkey, France, Spain, Tahiti, Bora-Bora, Moorea, and various U.S. locations for Bill's reunions of the USS *Davison* (a destroyer/minesweeper that was in service during World War II).

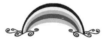

Volunteer Director of the Good Samaritan Food Ministry

While developing my business, I accepted the biblical challenge of loving others unselfishly and serving them. A very special person, who called himself Brother Michael, entered my life and became my mentor in serving the needy. For several years prior to his death in 1989, I supported his efforts, and after his death, tried to carry forth his service.

This food ministry was successful because of faithful volunteers who came to work and the faithful donors who stood by us. One recipient told a news reporter of the *Orange County Register*: "These people help us. We have no money for food sometimes, no money for the babies for Christmas. These people [provide] a happy time for us."[1]

I well remember those who helped me in this effort. Standing and holding hands in a circle around the serving tables, we each in turn would offer a prayer for the long line of men, women, and children patiently waiting for food and clothing. We came from different countries and races, and held different faiths. We did not speak a common language but served a common goal. God knows our names.

How often I have thanked God for allowing me to survive breast cancer and be in this place where love abounded among people who also knew about the adversities of life but who were not defeated. One could feel God's presence as we prayed together. The sound was beautiful, and peace filled the room.

When remembering that I was not even able to raise my hand above my head for several weeks after the mastectomy, and how radiation brought such fatigue, I truly realized how God had greatly blessed my life and our efforts to feed, clothe, and ease the burden of the needy.

The miracles of God's love are endless. I remember a well-groomed young man in his twenties, standing in line, holding a Bible. He said,

> "My name is Brent. You won't remember me, but one dark, cold morning in January, I hid between the trucks at the church. You saw me, didn't say anything about my having the DTs, asked if I was hungry and brought me food and hot coffee. You didn't preach to me, you just said, 'I love you and Jesus loves you; please take better care of yourself.' You brought me to the Lord. I am now a Christian, attend AA meetings, and I'm sober."

We embraced as I cried in gratitude. Although we never met again, my prayers for Brent will continue for as long as I live.

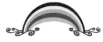

Love Creates the Emma Alberta School of English Literacy

Brother Michael's words kept resounding in my thoughts, "Why don't you come and teach my poor?" I answered that call to return to teaching. In 1991, after eighteen months and much prayer, I closed the food ministry because there were other food agencies available. I redirected my energy toward opening a non-profit school of English literacy named The Golden Rule Learning Center. In 1994, the school was renamed as The Emma Alberta School of English Literacy, in honor of my mother who had died at the age of eighty-nine.

The motivation to start our school seventeen years after my mastectomy was the children I encountered at The Good Samaritan Food Ministry. There they were: beautiful, black-eyed children staring up at me, clutching their mother's skirts, patiently waiting for bags of food and clothing. The sight broke my heart. These families were obviously mired in the cycle of poverty. I believed that the best way I could ultimately assist them over the long term was to encourage education for parents as well as their children.

Students of all races have been taught, from the ages of nine to seventy-two. They've come from Argentina, Bolivia, Brazil, Columbia, China, El Salvador, Guatemala, Italy, Japan, Lebanon, Mexico, Peru, Poland, Thailand, United States, Venezuela, Vietnam, and Yemen.

Many students have written letters of appreciation, such as a 1983 naturalized American citizen born in Mexico, who did not speak, write, or understand English prior to coming to our school:

> My three children are so proud of me because they also notice my improvement in English. I show them everything I do and read them my homework. They encourage me and say, 'Oh, Mom, we are so proud of you.' Dr. Marie Eckess teaches us confidence and self-esteem. I feel so comfortable in her class.

A Professor of Italian at UCSB wrote of her seventy-two-year-old mother:

> I just wanted to write and thank you for what your school has given my mother. Yes, I have noticed improvement in her English skills, but perhaps more importantly, I have seen my mother develop self-confidence in terms of her ability to communicate in English and in the worth of what she has to say. I am grateful that she has been able to attend your school in an environment that is encouraging and positive. She loves it,

looks forward to it, and is very grateful, as I am to all of you. Your school was a wonderful idea and is a generous and beautiful gift. Thank you.

Her mother was a brave Italian woman who had survived the bombing of her home in Italy during World War II, and who came to the United States as a war bride.

The Emma Alberta School of English Literacy continues to provide scholarships for educational opportunities to deserving students of all ages and races, regardless of where they study in the United States. Our scholarships have helped two adults graduate as certified nurses. Other individuals are studying for the following professions: cardiovascular technician, Catholic priest, nursing assistant, licensed practical nurse, and Christian chaplain, just to mention a few. All proceeds from the sale of this book, *Rainbow of Hope*, will be used to provide educational scholarships for the children whose mothers died from breast cancer.

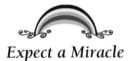

Expect a Miracle

Surrendering my life to the will of God resulted in the above positive services. These are just a few examples of God's many blessings in my life after breast cancer. My survival also made it possible for me to be at the bedside of my mother when she died, and to give the eulogy at her funeral. This was particularly precious to me as her only living child.

Another miracle of my life was surviving a noncancerous, double brain aneurysm in 1995, with my faculties intact and no visible bodily harm, except for another scar and skull impressions where they drilled three holes and cut facial muscles. I laughingly tell my friends that not only do I have a silicone friend sitting with me as I write this book, I literally have holes in my head with metal parts hiding under my hairline. I sometimes chuckle and shout, "Beam me up!"

I really can't find the words to describe the wonder I felt at God's allowing me to keep the use of my mind and eyes after the double brain aneurysm. I so want the remainder of my life to honor Him. Because of His mercy, my lifelong love of reading and learning continues.

Women of Faith and Courage

Reading the Bible has always been a source of encouragement to me. I identify with biblical women of faith and courage who had to undergo many tragedies in their lives, and I have repeatedly turned to them for inspiration. From this personal interest, I achieved another goal of developing and teaching a Bible study called "Women as Encouragers."

I undertook this study for personal growth and out of concern for the prevalent victim mentality in our society. I wanted to be a woman who encourages others to achieve their dreams. Further, I wanted to understand why I never seemed to be successful in helping those who give a "Yes, but . . ." excuse for refusing to assume personal responsibility. I saw this attitude in too many of the students who came to our school, as well as in a college class I recently attended to learn Spanish.

I acknowledge little patience for people who continue to accept and live a "Yes, but . . ." denial existence. Instead, I look for those positive people of courage and faith in my life and in literature who have the capacity to inspire, uplift, and encourage others as observed in their behavior while in the midst of adversity.

Bernice (43/44) spoke of a friend she loved who inspired her because of a "marvelous attitude" while waging a battle against breast cancer. My friend, Margaret, was such a person to me as she fought Lou Gehrig's Disease. My cousins, Emma and Helen, also inspire me because of their faith and courage.

As I write this book, my cousin Emma struggles against leukemia. Her sister, Helen, continues to bear the cross of deafness in one ear and constant ringing in her head, due to a noncancerous brain tumor removed twenty-seven years ago. These sisters offer the following coping suggestions:

- Put your faith in God: "Here I am Lord; thy will be done." God becomes a peaceful force of inner calm.
- Think positively. Life is nicer and easier with a positive attitude. Your family will be helped. The time you spend with a positive attitude will give you happy moments, even though there is intermittent pain.
- Keep yourself busy, one day at a time. Look at the beautiful things that surround you.
- Don't feel sorry for yourself. Look beyond the pain. Learn to live with it.
- Don't dwell on fear, as it never leaves us calm. Say to yourself, *I have to do it, so let's get on with it; the faster I get it over with, the better.*
- You have to find strength within yourself. No one can give it to you, it is from the Lord.
- If you are willing to overcome, you can. A lot has to do with personality, the inner core of who we are as a person. Some people can't stand even a minor illness, don't have the support of a family, and pity themselves so much that even friends finally turn away.
- Say to yourself, *I'm going to live with it day in and day out.*
- Learn to compensate for what you have lost. Don't think about it anymore.
- You must be the one to want to get better. At some place, you will be left on your own.
- Reach out to help others. People do need support, and many have no one.

These words of encouragement seem timeless and are similar to those spoken by the seventy women in 1974–1975. The greatest way to show appreciation for life is to live daily with acceptance and gratitude.

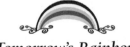

Tomorrow's Rainbow

Grace, a dear friend of mine who team-taught with me years ago, recently said, "You're always bubbling over with something new to do. You can get down sometimes, but most of the time you are bubbling over with a new project. I don't know what helps you to do that. I wish I knew so I could do it, too. I think it is wonderful. You keep your mind active, and you do things like the food ministry, your school, and now this book on surviving breast cancer. What's next?"

I trust that God will continue to show me what's next, and I strongly believe in the philosophy of Albert Schweitzer: "Seek always to do some good somewhere. You must give some time to your fellow man. For remember, you don't live in a world all your own."

With the help of God, I plan to live the remainder of my life with a positive attitude, honoring God by using my spiritual gifts in His service wherever He places me; sharing our bounty with friends, family, and strangers; and praising the Lord for His unending blessings, among the greatest of which is my life, and my devoted husband, Bill.

My fervent prayer is that God will soon send the world a cure for all cancer, particularly when I see children who have this disease. Until then, we must endure with faith. We must not surrender our hope. I am living proof, along with many others, that with the help of God, family, friends, and caregivers, we can and do survive breast cancer. We more than survive. We lead happy and productive lives. Together, we survivors keep hope alive until that glorious day when cancer no longer lives.

I will continue to search the horizon after a rainstorm where my heart will again see the seventy women of courage and faith I met in 1974–1975, and they will be looking and smiling back at me. I will forever see God's rainbow of hope.

"I will lift up mine eyes unto the hills,
from whence cometh my help.
My help cometh from the Lord."
—Psalm 121:1-2

ADDENDUM

A Few Important Questions to Ask

In order to understand the hopeful advancements that have been achieved by humanity in its fight against cancer, we need to have at least a cursory understanding of what has occurred in the past. We also need to keep ourselves informed as to promising research being conducted today.

What Do We Know about Cancer?

Scientific research tells us that cancer is not a monolithic disease, and there is no such thing as one type of breast cancer. We also know that cancer is not a new disease, but has plagued humanity for centuries. We are aware through historical documents that breast cancer was known by the early Egyptians and was most often treated by cauterizing the diseased tissue. There was no anesthesia.

Various explanations of what causes cancer have been given over the years. The Greek physician Caudius Galen (130–200 A.D.) said that melancholia was the culprit. Treatments included special diets, exorcism, and topical applications. During the Renaissance, mastectomy was recommended by the Flemish anatomist, Andreas Vesalius. It is reported that in 1700, Sister Barbier de l'Assumption, a nurse at L'Hotel Dieu Hospital in

Quebec City, Canada, underwent a mastectomy and lived for thirty years.

A major advancement in understanding cancer was made by Dr. LeDran (1685–1770), who recognized that breast cancer could spread to lymph nodes under the arm, resulting in a poor prognosis for survival. By the late 1800s, it was commonplace to do radical mastectomies and remove lymph nodes in hope of preventing the spread or recurrence of breast cancer. Today, more than 230 years after Dr. LeDran's discovery, physicians continue to use lymph node involvement as the basis for selecting patients for drug therapy trials.[1]

What Was Surgery Like Before Anesthesia?

A variety of approaches was used to dull the pain: narcotics made from a wide variety of plants such as marijuana, belladonna and jimsonweed; mesmerism or hypnosis; rubbing on counterirritants, such as stinging nettles; knocking patients into unconsciousness by hitting them in the jaw; by 1846, using opium, though it was not strong enough to kill the pain of surgery and had bad side effects; and using alcohol, which was likely to cause nausea, vomiting, and death because of the amount needed. Surgery was undertaken only as a last and desperate effort to save lives.[2]

When Was Anesthesia First Used?

A Boston dentist, William T. G. Morton, first used ether during surgery on October 16, 1846. A new era began for medicine, and anesthesia was declared the "greatest gift ever made to suffering humanity. . . . We have conquered pain."[3] Such men of science and their patients are among the many early courageous pioneers whose suffering has left a body of knowledge that benefits all future generations. Everyone who undergoes surgery owes these brave men and women a debt of gratitude.

Today, the discipline of anesthesiology is quite sophisticated and aided by computer-controlled environments.

"Ether has long been supplanted by newer and safer agents that allow more precise control of consciousness and result in fewer side effects like nausea. Anesthetic drugs that quickly disappear from the bloodstream allow many patients to go home within hours of certain surgical procedures."[4]

What Criteria Should We Use in Choosing a Mammogram Provider?

Since breast x-rays are particularly difficult to read, about 5 to 8 percent of women are called back for a follow-up mammogram. These false positives are due to weight change, medication, such as hormones, a breast injury, or dense breasts. Fatty tissues can mask tumors in their early stages. Being cautious, technicians call for follow-up exams, thus raising the costs of the procedure. The following guidelines are suggested in choosing a mammogram provider:

1. All mammography centers should be licensed by the State and accredited by the Food and Drug Administration.
2. Ask how many mammograms the radiologist reads a day. While there is no set number they should read in order to be proficient, "generally, the more you read the better you are," said Dr. Daniel Kopans, associate professor of radiology at Harvard Medical School.
3. Ask if the doctors do double readings on screening mammograms. A Swedish study showed that centers where two radiologists looked at each asymptomatic mammogram had a 15 percent higher cancer detection rate than a single evaluator.
4. Ask about the center's cancer detection rate. The national average is four to eight cancers per 1,000 women.[5]

The importance of choosing a qualified mammogram provider can be understood in light of a recent study:

Girls treated for childhood cancer with chest radiation are twenty times more likely to develop breast cancer later in life than other women, and they run an extremely high risk of getting it by their early twenties. Researchers suggested that after the first mammogram at twenty-five, childhood cancer survivors get one every three years until age forty. They also suggested annual breast exams by a doctor between puberty and twenty-five and two exams a year after that. After forty, they should have a mammogram every year.[6]

On June 25, 1998, the Food and Drug Administration approved the use of a computerized scanner, called ImageChecker, to double-check mammograms for signs of cancer that may have been missed by radiologists. For every eighty breast cancers mammograms diagnosed, the FDA estimate that about twenty are missed. Early detection is vital as there is a 90-percent chance of survival if the cancer is less than one centimeter in diameter.

The computer system analyzes mammography films that have been turned into digital signals. It compares each signal with its digitized database of cancerous mammograms, running about 300 to 400 million mathematical computations per film to search for subtle problems. The process takes three or four minutes. The signals are converted back into the mammogram image, with suspicious areas highlighted. Radiologists are expected to use the computer to double check their original interpretation of each mammogram. Interpretation errors account for about 10 percent of missed breast cancers; another 10 percent are overlooked because the cancers were too subtle.[7]

This is an exciting development but not foolproof because the FDA warns that the ImageChecker may cause more false alarms over benign lumps and has ordered the manufacturer, R2 Technology, Inc., to study this area of concern. Dr. Richard Reitherman, mammography chairman for the American Cancer Society of Southern California cautions that most U.S. mammograms "are not read by real experienced people."[8] Approximately thirty million American women have mammograms each year.

Where Can We Find a Good Prosthesis?

The improvements made in prosthesis since 1974–1975 are to be commended. Breast forms can be made from foam, fiberfill, or silicone. There is now a greater variety of lighter-weight shapes and sizes in silicone that can either be worn in your bra or attached directly to your chest wall. We have choices of select colors to match our skin tone. The choice of a prosthesis is truly individual, depending upon lifestyle and breast size.

In purchasing, we have the option of going to a department store, ordering from various companies over the Internet, or going to a store that specializes in medical and surgical supplies and who have certified fitters (my personal choice).

All these options mean nothing if we are not properly fitted, no matter how kind and understanding the salesperson may be. A prosthesis that proves to be too large or too small or ill-fitted in any way simply compounds our feelings of loss and frustration. Proper fitting improves posture and reduces back pain and shoulder aches from tight bra straps. I currently wear a silicone Amoena made by Coloplast Corporation, which also carries a line of postmastectomy brassieres, swimsuits, and therapeutic skin-care products.

I believe that women need to work with a certified fitter who also has empathy rather than discomfort when helping us. Denise (56/57) had said, "The salesclerk was more embarrassed than I was. I was more embarrassed for the clerk than for myself."

I have had similar experiences over the years, but not since I chose a certified fitter who also deals with numerous other medical and surgical needs. As a trained professional, she has perspective and shows genuine empathy because she sees other people with various prosthesis requirements, resulting from strokes, surgery, motor accidents, and pregnancy. My certified fitter has numerous dedicated years of experience and knowledge.

I recently asked her what she would like women to know about the prosthesis and women's attitudes about the mastectomy. She responded, "If your prosthesis is properly fitted, you don't need any special garments or clothing. Women who come in crying and saying, 'Dear Lord, what's happening to me?' are now pushing up daisies. The ones who come in with a happy heart are still with me. Your body is a temple of the Lord. Be grateful for what you have."

What Coverage Is Provided by Insurance Carriers for the Prosthesis?

Medicare covers breast forms and mastectomy bras. The dollar amount varies, but usually ranges in price from $200 to $250 for a silicone breast prosthesis, to $20 to $30 for a mastectomy bra. Most private insurers include breast forms in their basic benefit package, but coverage varies by company and plan. Some companies cover a breast form yearly, while others may cover only one per lifetime after the insured has paid a deductible and copayment. It is important to ask your insurance carrier what coverage is provided.

I believe it is vitally important to a woman's physical and emotional well-being to be fitted properly and comfortably, regardless of the amount of insurance coverage.

What Coverage Is Provided by Insurance Carriers for Postmastectomy Breast Reconstruction, Including Work on the Remaining Breast to Restore Symmetry?

Some insurers still consider such surgery to be "cosmetic" and not a medical necessity. They lump postmastectomy breast reconstruction with nose jobs, tummy tucks, face lifts, liposuction, breast enlargements, breast reductions, and other such plastic surgery done to refine nature for the beauty-conscious.

> Some plans are denying or fighting claims for reconstructive surgery for children with facial deformities, women who have had mastectomies, and accident victims with scars and burns . . . . Insurers say they have been forced to take a tough line on plastic surgery because of years of abuse by some doctors and patients seeking coverage for strictly vanity work. Moreover, insurers say that they will pay for truly corrective work but that it isn't their responsibility to finance endless improvements. Joseph Berman, chief medical officer for Anthem Blue Cross & Blue Shield in Mason, Ohio, asks, 'Is society prepared to pay for beauty? I don't think our mission is to make all kids beautiful. But we would like to make them as normal as we can.'[9]

We live in a society that preaches the extreme of body-perfect which leads to a Ponce de Leon Complex that often becomes a vanity obsession. This obsession can be seen in so many of our young girls who become anorexic and bulimic out of fear of gaining weight, and in women who have repeated plastic surgery in search of yesterday's youth but whose satisfaction with temporary results is fleeting.

How can we go to the other extreme by refusing adequate insurance coverage for reconstructive surgery for children born with facial deformities, women with mastectomies, and accident victims with scars and burns? After all, a woman wanting to have the wrinkles removed from her forehead because she wants to appear younger cannot be compared to a woman who has lost her breast to cancer.

I believe that people reasoning together can develop insurance policies that will cover medical expenses arising from bodily harm caused by birth defects, disease, and accident. Questing for yesterday's youth through vanity surgery is a separate issue.

Currently, congress is considering several pending bills that would require insurers to pay for postmastectomy breast reconstruction, to include surgery on the remaining breast in order to restore symmetry. Although such laws exist in over half the States, many self-insured plans are exempt.

How Can We Find Out about Promising Research That May Cure Cancer?

Using the age-old methods of visiting libraries, reading newspapers and magazines, watching educational programs on TV, and contacting such agencies as the American Cancer Society, all remain valuable sources. I highly recommend two books: *Estrogen and Breast Cancer: A Warning to Women* by Carol Ann Rinzler, and *Breast Care Options for the 1990s* by Paul Kuehn, M.D.

Computer access to the Internet is truly a marvel in gathering information. Data concerning cancer surgery options, radiation, and chemotherapy can be accessed from Memorial Sloan-Kettering Cancer Center (web site: http://www.mskcc.org): from Mayo Health Oasis (web site: http://www.mayohealth.org): from the National Cancer Institute (web site: http://rex.nci.nih.gov), among many others. However, we must still use cautious discernment in interpreting what we are told. The following examples prove this point.

What Promising Research Is Currently Underway?

We are told of an *alternative medicine* to chemotherapy being used in Italy by Dr. Luigi Di Bellia, which is a clinically untested cocktail of hormones and vitamins. Several cancer physicians caution cancer patients not to abandon the known treatments of chemotherapy and radiation as Dr. Di Bellia's alternative medicine is not proven even though many patients in Italy swear by his treatment. Italy has decided to run clinical trials and is expected to announce the results soon.[10]

Many so-called *designer hormone drugs* are being introduced. Before winning government approval, new drugs first are tested on animals then go through three phases of human testing: phase I tests for safety in humans; phase II tests for effectiveness in a small number of people; and phase III then uses the drugs on a large number of people, testing for both effectiveness and safety in humans.

Drugs often have side effects and can include increased risks leading to cancer in the uterine lining and breast, as well as blood clots in the lungs. Such risks may offset the benefits. "You need to be clear about what the risks are so you're not trading one disease for another," said Georgia Wiesner, a medical director at the Center for Human Genetics at University Hospital, Cleveland. In agreement with this advice is Cindy Pearson, executive director of the National Women's Health Network: "Women can decide how they want to play the odds, but they need to know the odds."[11]

Two drugs, *endostatin* and *angiostatin*, used by Dr. Moses Judah Folkman of Boston's Children's Hospital, have successfully make tumors disappear and not return in mice. Dr. Folkman's revolutionary discovery is that "tumor cells must secrete some natural compound to induce blood vessels to sprout tiny capillaries. Without the come-hither molecule, capillaries do not connect to a tumor; without a custom-grown blood supply, the tumor stays dormant."[12] As far back as 1971, when President Richard Nixon called for a war on cancer, Dr. Folkman met with hostility, rejection, and ridicule from colleagues about his theory. Today, he has sparked hope in the hearts of many.

"We are driven by hope," said Dr. Jerome Groopman, a cancer researcher at the Harvard Medical School, "but a sober scientist waits for the data."[13] Even Dr. Folkman is cautious about the drugs' promise and says that until the drugs are used on humans, predictions are dangerous.

> In an interview, Folkman said the National Cancer Institute hopes to test the new drugs, called angiostatin and endostatin, on about thirty adults with brain, lung, and other cancers in whom all other treatments have failed. Folkman said a cancer institute facility in Frederick, Maryland, planned to produce just enough (of the two drugs) for a small number of patients. So far they're right on schedule for December or the first of the year. That's our hope. [14]

Dr. Folkman's initial rejection by his colleagues reminds me of Dr. Ignaz Semmelweis, a seventeenth-century doctor, who worked in a hospital in Vienna that had an extremely high mortality in pregnant women due to puerperal fever. "It was Ignaz Semmelweis who showed that the infective material that caused this disease was conveyed by the hands of the doctors and medical students from the autopsy room to the expectant mother. He was virtually laughed out of the profession, and ended his days in a lunatic asylum."[15]

Today, Dr. Semmelweis is honored because of his call to cleanliness as a necessity to combat disease. We know that we can help stop the spread of disease simply by washing our hands. Thus, what was scorned in the seventeenth century as unsound medical practice is now thoroughly accepted in our twentieth century. Knowledge keeps advancing.

The excitement generated by the suggestion of yet another possible cure for cancer continues to exist side-by-side with disbelief and admonition for caution because of past failed expectations. Due to new gene-based drugs today, J. Michael Bishop, a Nobel laureate in cancer research says, "For the first time in my life, I believe we will eventually be able to conquer cancer."[16]

Another exciting development is the **new procedure where surgeons remove only one lymph node, the sentinel node,** where cancer cells travel first from the breast tumor.

Today more breast cancers are being diagnosed at an early stage, thanks to improved screening. But in 80 percent of these patients, axillary node dissection shows that the lymph nodes are cancer free. The new procedure of taking only the sentinel node can be performed on patients who opt either for lumpectomy or mastectomy, but is most effective if a woman's tumor is two centimeters (2.54 cm. = 1 inch) or less in size. Thus the importance of early detection. Besides reducing the chance of developing lymphedema, sentinel node biopsy offers other benefits: it can be done under local anesthesia, does not require an overnight hospital stay, decreases the risk of surgical complications, and results in lower medical costs.[17]

I lament that too many minority women are not having follow-up treatment as shown in the results of a recent study by Dr. Roshan Bastani, associate professor of public health at the University of California, Los Angeles, and an expert in cancer and minorities:

> When a breast abnormality was diagnosed in white women, nearly 99 percent visited their doctors for follow-up treatment. But among minority women in her study, who were primarily black and Hispanic but included a small number of Asians, only 75 percent sought follow-up care. 'Part of this has to do with attitudes,' Dr. Bastani said, 'like, it will go away, or I don't have sick leave, so if I go in for this, I'm going to lose a day's pay. Even when minorities have good insurance, they do not always take advantage of it.'[18]

My caution to women of all races is that until a miracle cure for cancer actually occurs, we must all continue to concentrate on early detection through monthly breast self-examinations, yearly clinical examinations, and yearly mammograms as the proven successful methods to fight all forms of cancer. The attitude of fear and denial often results in death.

GLOSSARY

adenocarcinoma. Cancer that starts in the glandular tissue, such as in the lobules or ducts of the breast.

adrenalectomy. The removal of one or both adrenal glands located near each kidney that produce female hormones (estrogens and progesterone).

advanced cancer. A stage of cancer in which the disease has spread from the primary site to other parts of the body. When the cancer has spread only to the surrounding areas, it is called locally advanced. If it has spread further by traveling through the network of lymph glands (lymphatics) or in the bloodstream, it is called metastatic.

antiestrogen. A substance (for example, the drug taxmoxifen) that blocks the effects of estrogen on tumors. Antiestrogens are used to treat breast cancers that depend on estrogen for growth.

areola. The dark area of flesh that surrounds the nipple of the breast.

asymptomatic. To be without noticeable symptoms of disease. Many cancers can develop and grow without producing symptoms, especially in the early stages. Screening tests, such as mammography, try to discover developing cancers at the asymptomatic stage, when the chances for cure are usually highest.

axillary dissection. A surgical procedure in which the lymph nodes in the armpit (axillary nodes) are removed and examined to find out if breast cancer has spread to those nodes.

benign. Not cancer; not malignant. The main types of benign breast problems are fibroadenomas and fibrocystic changes.

bilateral. Affecting both sides of the body; for example, bilateral breast cancer is cancer occurring in both breasts at the same time (synchronous) or at different times (metachronous).

biopsy. A procedure in which tissue samples are removed from the body for examination of their appearance under a microscope to find out if cancer or other abnormal cells are present. A biopsy can be done with a needle or by surgery.

bone scan. An imaging method that gives important information about the growth and health of bones, including the location of cancer that may have spread to the bones. It can be done as an outpatient procedure and is painless, except for the needle stick when a low-dose radioactive substance is injected into a vein. Images are taken to see where the radioactivity accumulates, indicating an abnormality.

BRCA1 and **BRCA2.** Genes which, when damaged or mutated, places a woman at greater risk of developing breast/or ovarian cancer.

breast cancer. Cancer that starts in the breast. The main types of breast cancer are ductal carcinoma in situ, invasive ductal carcinoma, lobular carcinoma in situ, invasive lobular carcinoma, medullary carcinoma, and Paget's disease of the nipple.

breast implant. A manufactured sac that is filled with silicone gel (a synthetic material) or saline (sterile saltwater). The sac is surgically inserted to increase breast size or restore the contour of a breast after mastectomy. Because of concern about possible (but as yet unproven) side effects of silicone, silicone implants are presently available only to women who agree to participate in a clinical trial in which side effects are carefully monitored.

breast reconstruction. Surgery that rebuilds the breast contour after mastectomy. A breast implant or the woman's own tissue provides the contour. If desired, the nipple and areola may also be re-created. Reconstruction can be done at the time of mastectomy or any time later.

breast self-exam (BSE). A technique of checking one's own breasts for lumps or suspicious changes. The method is recommended for all women over age 20, to be done once a month, usually at a time other than the days before, during, or immediately after her menstrual period.

calcifications. Tiny calcium deposits within the breast, singly or in clusters, often found by mammography. These are also called microcalcifications. They are a sign of change within the breast that may be monitored by additional, periodic mammograms, or by immediate or delayed biopsy. They may be caused by breast cancer or by benign breast conditions.

cancer cell. A cell that divides and reproduces abnormally and can spread throughout the body.

carcinoma. A malignant tumor that begins in the lining layer (epithelial cells) of organs. At least 80 percent of all cancers are carcinomas, and almost all breast cancers are carcinomas.

carcinoma in situ. An early stage of cancer, in which the tumor is still only in the structures of the organ where it first developed, and the disease has not invaded other parts of the organ or spread (metastasized). Most in situ carcinomas are highly curable.

chemotherapy. Treatment with drugs to destroy cancer cells. Chemotherapy is often used in addition to surgery or radiation to treat cancer when metastasis is proven or suspected, when the cancer has come back (recurred), or when there is a strong likelihood that the cancer could recur.

cyst. A fluid-filled mass that is usually benign. The fluid can be removed for analysis. (needle aspiration).

dimpling. A pucker or indentation of the skin on the breast may be a sign of cancer.

duct: A hollow passage for gland secretions. In the breast, a passage through which milk passes from the lobule (which makes the milk) to the nipple.

edema. Build-up of fluid in the tissues, resulting in swelling. Edema of the arm can occur after radical mastectomy, axillary dissection of lymph nodes, or radiation therapy.

estrogen. A female sex hormone produced primarily by the ovaries, and in smaller amounts by the adrenal cortex. In breast cancer, estrogen may promote the growth of cancer cells.

estrogen replacement therapy (ERT). The use of exogenous estrogen (estrogen not produced by the body; estrogen from other sources) after the body has ceased to produce it because of natural or induced menopause. This type of hormone therapy is often prescribed to alleviate symptoms of menopause and has been shown to provide protective effects against heart disease and osteoporosis in postmenopausal women. Since estrogen nourishes some types of breast cancer, scientists are working on the question of whether estrogen replacement therapy increases breast cancer risk.

fat necrosis. The death of fat cells, usually following injury. Fat necrosis is a benign condition, but it can cause a breast lump, pulling of the skin, or skin changes that can be confused with breast cancer.

fibroadenoma. A type of benign breast tumor composed of fibrous tissue and glandular tissue. On clinical examination or breast self-examination, it usually feels like a firm, round, smooth lump. These usually occur in young women.

fibrocystic changes. A term that describes certain benign changes in the breast; also called fibrocystic disease. Symptoms of this condition are breast swelling or pain. Signs that a health care professional can observe on clinical breast examination are the nodularity (nodules), lumpiness, and sometimes, nipple discharge. Because these signs sometimes mimic breast cancer, diagnostic mammography or microscopic examination of breast tissue may be needed to show that there is no cancer.

internal mammary nodes. Lymph nodes beneath the breast bone on each side. Some breast cancers may spread to these nodes.

lobular carcinoma in situ (LCIS). A very early type of breast cancer that develops within the milk-producing glands (lobules) of the breast and does not penetrate the wall of the lobules. Researchers think that most cases of lobular carcinoma in situ do not progress to invasive lobular cancer. However, having this type of cancer places a woman at increased risk of developing an invasive breast cancer later in life. For this reason, it's important for women with lobular carcinoma in situ to have a physical examination three times a year and an annual mammogram.

localized breast cancer. A cancer that started in the breast and is confined to the breast.

lumpectomy. Surgery to remove the breast tumor and a small amount of surrounding normal tissue.

lymph. Clear fluid that passes within the lymphatic system and contains cells known as lymphocytes. These cells are important in fighting infections and may also have a role in fighting cancer.

lymph nodes. Small bean-shaped collections of immune system tissue such as lymphocytes, located along lymphatic vessels. They remove waste and fluids from lymph and help fight infections. Also called lymph glands.

lymphedema. Swelling in the arm caused by excess fluid that collects after lymph nodes and vessels are removed by surgery or treated by radiation. This condition is usually painful and can be persistent.

malignant tumor. A mass of cancer cells that may invade surrounding tissues or spread (metastasize) to distant areas of the body.

mammogram, mammography. An x-ray of the breast; the principal method of detecting breast cancer in women over forty. A mammogram can show a developing breast tumor before it is large enough to be felt by a woman or even by a highly skilled health care professional. Screening mammography is used for early detection of breast cancer without any breast symptoms. Diagnostic mammography is used to help characterize breast masses or determine the cause of other breast symptoms.

mastectomy. Surgery to remove all or part of the breast and sometimes other tissue. (1) Extended radical mastectomy removes the breast, skin, nipple, areola, chest muscles (pectoral major and minor), and all axillary and internal mammary lymph nodes on the same side. (2) Halsted radical mastectomy removes the breast, skin, nipple, both pectoral muscles, and all axillary lymph nodes on the same side. (3) Modified radical mastectomy removes the breast, skin, nipple, areola, and most of the axillary lymph nodes on the same side, leaving the chest muscles intact. (4) Partial mastectomy removes less than the whole breast, taking only part of the breast in which the cancer occurs and a margin of healthy breast tissue surrounding the tissue. (5) Subcutaneous mastectomy is surgery to remove internal breast tissue. The nipple and skin are left intact.

(6) Prophylactic mastectomy is a subcutaneous mastectomy done before any evidence of cancer can be found, for the purpose of preventing cancer. This procedure is sometimes recommended for women at very high risk of breast cancer. (7) Quadrantectomy is a partial mastectomy in which the quarter of the breast that contains a tumor is removed. (8) Segmental mastectomy is a partial mastectomy. (9) Simple mastectomy or total mastectomy removes only the breast and areola.

mastitis. Inflammation or infection of the breast.

metastasis. The spread of cancer cells to distant areas of the body by way of the lymph system or bloodstream.

needle aspiration. A type of needle biopsy. Removal of fluid from a cyst or cells from a tumor. In this procedure, a needle and syringe (like those used to give injections) is used to pierce the skin, reach the cyst or tumor, and with suction, draw up (aspirate) specimens for biopsy analysis. If the needle is thin, the procedure is called a fine needle aspiration.

needle biopsy. Removal of fluid, cells, or tissue with a needle for examination under a microscope. There are two types: fine needle aspiration (also called FNA or needle aspiration) and core biopsy. FNA uses a thin needle, a core needle is thicker to remove a cylindrical sample of tissues from a tumor.

oncologist. A doctor who is specially trained in the diagnosis and treatment of cancer. Medical oncologists specialize in the use of chemotherapy and other drugs to treat cancer. Radiation oncologists specialize in the use of x rays (radiation) to kill tumors.

oophorectomy. Surgery to remove the ovaries.

osteoporosis. Breakdown of bone, resulting in diminished bone mass and reduced bone strength. Osteoporosis can cause pain, deformity (especially of the spine), fractures (broken bones). This condition is common among postmenopausal women.

pathologist. A physician who specializes in diagnosis and classification of diseases by laboratory tests (such as examination of tissue and cells under a microscope). The pathologist determines whether a lump is benign or cancerous.

pectoral muscles. Muscles attached to the front of the chest wall and upper arms. The larger group is called pectoralis major, and a smaller group is called pectoralis minor. Because these muscles are next to the breast, breast cancer may sometimes spread to the pectoral muscles.

prognosis. A prediction of the course of disease; the outlook for the cure of the patient. For example, women with breast cancer that was detected early and received prompt treatment have a good prognosis.

prosthesis. An artificial form, such as a breast prosthesis, that can be worn under the clothing after a mastectomy. (Plural: prostheses.)

Reach to Recovery. A visitation program of the American Cancer Society for women who have a personal concern about breast cancer. Carefully selected and trained volunteers who have successfully adjusted to breast cancer and its treatment provide information and support to women newly diagnosed with the disease.

recurrence. Cancer that has come back after treatment. (1) Local recurrence is at the same site as the original cancer. (2) Regional recurrence is in the lymph nodes near the site of origin. (3) Distant recurrence is in organs or tissues further from the original site than the regional lymph nodes (such as the lungs, liver, bone marrow, or brain). (4) Metastasis means that the disease has recurred at a distant site.

remission. Complete or partial disappearance of the signs and symptoms of cancer in response to treatment; the period during which a disease is under control. A remission may not be a cure.

saline. Saltwater solution.

sarcoma. A malignant tumor growing from connective tissues, such as cartilage, fat, muscle, or bone. Several types of sarcoma (such as angiosarcoma, liposarcoma, and malignant phylloides tumor) can develop in the breast, and they differ in their prognosis.

side effects. Unwanted effects of treatment, such as hair loss caused by chemotherapy, and fatigue caused by radiation therapy.

silicone gel. Synthetic material used in breast implants because of its flexibility, strength, and texture, which is similar to the texture of the natural breast. Silicone gel breast implants are available for women who have had breast cancer surgery, but only if they participate in a clinical trial.

staging. The process of determining and describing the extent of cancer. Staging of breast cancer is based on the size of the tumor, whether regional axillary lymph nodes are involved, and whether distant spread (metastasis) has occurred. Knowing the stage at diagnosis is essential in selecting the best treatment and predicting a patient's outlook for survival.

stereotactic needle biopsy. A method of needle biopsy that is useful in some cases in which calcifications or a mass can be seen on mammogram but cannot be located by touch. Computerized equipment maps the location of the mass and this is used as a guide for the placement of the needle.

survival rate. The percentage of people who live a certain period of time. For example, the five-year survival rate for women with localized breast cancer (including all women living five years after diagnosis, whether the patient was in remission, disease-free, or under treatment) was 78 percent in the 1940s, but in the 1990s, it is over 97 percent.

tamoxifen (brand name: Nolvadex). A drug that blocks estrogen; an antiestrogen drug. Blocking estrogen is desirable in some cases of breast cancer because estrogen promotes their growth.

tumor. A lump or mass which has formed due to excessive accumulation of abnormal cells: can be benign (noncancerous) or malignant (cancerous).

x-rays. One form of radiation that can, at low levels, produce an image of the body on film and at high levels, can destroy cancer cells.

Glossary developed by the American Cancer Society
http://www.cancer.org/bcn/bcdict.html

ENDNOTES

Chapter 2: Early Detection Saves Lives

1. "What is Cancer?" American Cancer Society: Breast Cancer Network (1998)Internet: http://www.cancer.org/bcn/info/brcancer.html

2. "Can Breast Cancer Be Found Early?" American Cancer Society (1998) Internet: http://www.cancer.org/bcn/info/brearly.html

3. "Breast Self-Examination," American Cancer Society brochure, (1998)

4. "What Are the Key Statistics about Breast Cancer?" *Ibid.* Internet: http://www.cancer.org/bcn/info/brstats.html

5. "Risk Factors of Cancer," UMDNJ-University Hospital, (1998) Internet: http://www.umdnj.edu/univhosp/b1.html

6. *Ibid.*

7. "What Are the Risk Factors for Breast Cancer?" American Cancer Society, (1998) Internet: http://www.cancer.org/bcn/info/brrisk.html

8. "Anti-osteoporosis drug rivals estrogen, new study concludes." *The Orange County Register*, Health and Science, February 19, 1998.

9. Haas, Jane Glenn, "Doctor offers another angle on the estrogen question." *Ibid.*, March 1998

10. Steptoe, A. and Wardle, J. "What the experts think: a European survey of expert opinion about the influence of lifestyle on health." *European Journal of Epidemiology,* 4/10/94

11. Alexander, Duane, MD, Director. "Endometriosis 2000 meeting focuses on research agenda." *NICHD Research Reports,* July 1995.

12. Gray, Dr. Ron. "Abortion and Cancer," *Johns Hopkins Health NewsFeed* (1998) Internet: http://hopkins.med.jhu.edu/ NewsMedia/hnf/HNF_428.HTM

13. Brind, Dr. Joel, Ph.D. "Rotten in Denmark." (1997). Internet: http://www.abortioncancer.com.denmark.htm

14. Willke, J. C., MD. "The deadly after-effect of abortion: breast cancer." Roe v. Wade—25 years of life denied. (1998) Internet: http://www.profile.org/rvw/women6.html

15. "Abortion and Breast Cancer." *The New England Journal of Medicine.* Health News, 11/5/96. Internet: http://www. healthnet.ivi.com/hnews/9611/htm/politic.htm

16. "Study: Gene defects tied to breast cancer rarer than thought." *The Orange County Register Newspaper.* March 25, 1998.

17. "Mixed results in study of pre-emptive surgery." *The Orange County Register Newspaper.* Health and Science, March 7, 1998.

18. "How is Breast Cancer diagnosed?" American Cancer Society: Breast Cancer Network. (1998), Internet: http:// www.cancer.org/bcn/info/brdiagno.html

19. *Ibid.*

20. "Diagnosis of Breast Cancer." Memorial Sloan-Kettering Cancer Center (1998) Internet: http://www.mskcc.org/ document/wicbrst3.htm

21. *The Philosophy of Civilization.* NY: Macmillan, Paperback Edition, 1960, pp. 310-311.

Chapter 3: Selecting the Right Doctors

1. Hatcher, C., Brooks L., and Love C. "Breast cancer and silicone implants: psychological consequences for women." *Journal of the National Cancer Institute.* Sept. 1, 1993.

2. Walker Craig M., M.D., Medical Director, Cardiovascular Institute of the South. "Heart guidelines dispute underscores

importance of doctor selection." Internet: http://www.
cardio.com/article/guidelns.htm

3. "Group names troubled doctors." *The Orange County Register.*
March 5, 1998.

4. Burling, Stacey. "How do you know your doctor is good?"
The Orange County Register. April 12, 1998.

5. *Ibid.*

6. Kowalczyk, Liz. "Study examines doctors' bedside manner."
The Orange County Register. March 19, 1998.

7. *Ibid.*

8. Weintraub, Daniel M., and Nicolosi, Michelle. "Deal made
on HMO referrals." *The Orange County Register.* March 19,
1998.

9. *Ibid.*

Chapter 4: Surgery and Treatment

1. "How is Breast Cancer Treated?" American Cancer Society:
Breast Cancer Network Internet: http://www.cancer.org/
bcn/info/brtreat.html

2. *Ibid.*

3. Pilgrim, Ina. *The Topic of Cancer.* Thomas Y. Crowell
Company: NY, 1974.

Chapter 5: Badge of Courage

1. Hurny C, Bernard J, Bacchi M, van Wegberg B, Tomamichel
M, Seik U, Coates A, Castiglione M, Goldhirsch A, and Senn
HJ, et. al. "The Perceived Adjustment to Chronic Illness
Scale (PACIS): a global indicator of coping for operable
breast cancer patients in clinical trials." Swiss Group for
Clinical Cancer Research (SAKK) and the International
Breast Cancer Study Group (IBCSB). *Supportive Care in
Cancer,* July 1, 1993: 200-8.

Chapter 7: Husband Reactions

1. Baider, L. "Psychological intervention with couples after mastectomy," *Supportive Care in Cancer.* 1995 July, 3: 239-43.

Chapter 9: Implants and Prosthesis

1. Kuehn, Paul, M.D. *Breast Care Options for the 1990's*. South Windsor, CT: Newmark Publishing Company, 1991, p. 153.
2. *Ibid.*, pgs. 141, 144, 157.
3. Uthman, Ed, M.D. "On Breast Implant Hysteria," Internet: http://www.neosoft.com/uthman/rants/on_implant_hysteria.html Rant originally posted March 31, 1996.
4. Burton, Thomas M. "Dow Corning Has $4.4 Billion Plan on Chapter 11 and Implant Claims." *The Wall Street Journal.* February 18, 1998.

Chapter 13: God's Rainbow of Hope

1. "Marcus Aurelius, Meditation." *Marcus Aurelius and His Times*, Printed in U.S.A.: Walter J. Black, Inc., 1945.
2. Kubler-Ross, Elisabeth, M.D. *Questions and Answers on Death and Dying*. N.Y. and London: Macmillan Publishing Co., Inc., and Collier Macmillan Publishers, 1974.

Chapter 14: Twenty-Five Years of Survival

1. Miller, Jeffrey. "Samaritan's mission is to fill void, help needy." *The Orange County Register.* December 26, 1990.

Addendum

1. "BCSC" Breast Cancer History (1/2)", *BCSC*, Internet: http://www.bcse.ca/historyl.html
2. Sullivan, John T., M.D. "Surgery before anesthesia," *MGH Neurosurgery.* Internet: http://neurosurgery.mgh.harvard.edu/History/beforeth.htm
3. "Medicine's greatest gift." *MGH Neurosurgery.* Internet: http://neurosurgery.mgh.harvard.edu/History/gift.htm
4. "The evolution of ether: Today's anesthesiology." *MGH Neurosurgery.* Internet: http://neurosurgery.mgh.harvard.edu/History/evolve.htm
5. Gordon, Debra. "Follow-up common for breast screenings." *The Orange County Register.* April 18, 1998.

6. Meyer, Tara. "Girls treated for childhood cancer more likely to develop it again later." The Associated Press, *The Orange County Register*, February 13, 1998.

7. Sharpe, Rochelle. "Computer System to Detect Cancer Gets FDA Approval." *The Wall Street Journal*. June 30, 1998.

8. Neergaard, Lauran. "FDA approves device to check mammograms." The Associated Press, *The Orange County Register*. June 30, 1998.

9. Jeffrey, Nancy Ann. "Corrective or Cosmetic? Plastic Surgery Stirs a Debate." *The Wall Street Journal*. June 25, 1998.

10. Wakin, Daniel J. "Italy astir over doctor's cancer treatment." The Associated Press, *The Orange County Register*. February 4, 1998.

11. Winslow, Ron. "Pill to Prevent Breast Cancer Viewed Warily." *The Wall Street Journal*, 1998.

12. Kalb, Claudia, and Begley, Sharon. "One man's quest to cure cancer." *Newsweek*. May 18, 1998.

13. Kolata, Gina. "2 drugs may be cancer's nemesis." *The New York Times, The Orange County Register*. May 3, 1998.

14. Crewdson, John. "Touted cancer drugs may be tested on terminal patients." *Chicago Tribune, The Orange County Register*. May 17, 1998.

15. Pilgrim, Ira. *The Topic of Cancer*. N.Y.: Thomas Y. Crowell Company, 1974.

16. Langreth, Robert. "Arsenal of Hope." *The Wall Street Journal, The Orange County Register*. May 10, 1998.

17. "Sentinel node biopsy." Memorial Sloan-Kettering Cancer Center. Internet: http://www.mskcc.org

18. Stolberg, Sheryl Gay. "Light shed on minorities, cancer." *The New York Times, The Orange County Register*. March 14, 1998.

To order additional copies of

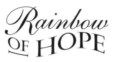

Rainbow
OF HOPE

send $15.95 plus $4.95 shipping
and handling to

Books, Etc.
PO Box 1406
Mukilteo, WA 98275

or have your credit card ready
and call

(800) 917-BOOK

You may also order directly from the
author. Please make checks payable to

Emma Alberta School
1048 Irvine Ave. #438
Newport Beach, CA 92660